SOTHIS PRESS

Sothis Press aims to completely reimagine the public domain book with an emphasis on universal access to captivatingly designed print editions. We believe that technology will enable every single book ever published to be perpetually accessible in beautiful print form. Sothis is beauty in ubiquity.

www.sothis.press
1 Waterhouse Square, London, EC1N 2ST

The Married Woman's Private Medical Companion

Embracing the Treatment of Menstruation, or Monthly Turns, During Their Stoppage, Irregularity, or Entire Suppression; Pregnancy, and How It May Be Determined; With the Treatment of Its Various Diseases; Discovery to Prevent Pregnancy

A. M. Mauriceau

SOTHIS PRESS

ISBN 978-1-83548-402-9

PREGNACY,

AND

HOW IT MAY BE DETERMINED;

WITH THE TREATMENT OF ITS VARIOUS DISEASES.

DISCOVERY TO

PREVENT PREGNACY;

THE GREAT AND IMPORTANT NECESSITY WHERE MALFORMATION OR INABILITY EXISTS TO GIVE BIRTH.

TO PREVENT MISCARRIAGE OR ABORTION

WHEN PROPER AND NECESSARY

TO EFFECT MISCARRIAGE.

WHEN ATTENDED WITH ENTIRE SAFETY.

CA

OR STERILITY.

BY DR. A. M. MAURICEAU
Professor of Diseases of Women.

Office, 129 Liberty steert.

NEW YORK:
1855.

PREFACE.

The "Introduction" in the succeeding pages, being amply explanatory, but few prefatory words will suffice. The object and intention of the work is manifest and self-evident.

It is to extend to every female, whether wife, mother or daughter, such information as will best qualify her to judge of her own maladies, and, having ascertained their existence, apply the proper remedies.

From these pages she will learn the causes, the symptoms and the remedies, for such complaints to which she may be liable, the nature of which she may not desire to impart to another.

Whether married or unmarried, she can, from these pages, compare her own symptoms with those described, and act in accordance with the mode of treatment prescribed. She will thereby be exempt from those doubts, perplexities and anxieties, which arise from nature contemplates an important change, the "Married Woman's Private Medical Companion" contains instructions of such paramount importance, as to embrace the present happiness and future welfare of each.

One word in conclusion. It is not pretended that the concentration of the results of medical research emanates from *one* author, for be he ever so versed in medical science, he would come far, far short of so herculean a task. It is, therefore, necessarily derived from authors on medical and physiological sciences, of great acquirements and distinguished celebrity.

It hardly need be added that great labour has been encountered in the preparation of a work of this nature, as the most reliable and correct sources have been availed of.

THE AUTHOR.

NOTICE.

To prevent confusion, those writing to *Dr. A. M. Mauriceau* will please be particular in giving their address and directions, specifying Town or Village, County and State.

INDEX.

		PAGE.
ABORTION—		
"	Symptoms of,	169
"	Causes of,	171
"	Treatment of,	171
"	Prevention of,	175
	When dangerous,	168
"	When necessary to effect,	177
"	When attended with no danger,	169
AFTER PAINS—		
"	Causes of,	203
"	Treatment of,	204
AFTER BIRTH—		
"	Caution respecting,	199
"	Mode of extracting,	199
ARTIFICIAL DELIVERY,		180
BARRENNESS, OR STERILITY—		223
"	Causes of,	225
"	Treatment of,	230
"	Remedy for,	232
CONCEPTION—(See Pregnancy)		36
"	Signs of,	37
"	Prevention of (See Pregnancy),	104
CHILDREN—Management of,		210
CONCLUDING REMARKS,		237
DELIVERY—Artificial,		180
DISEASES OF PREGNANCY,		61
	Desomeaux's Prevention to Pregnancy,	142
FALSE PAINS IN PREGNANCY,		187
FALSE Conception,		30
FAINTING, during Pregnancy,		87
"	Treatment of,	87

PAGE.
FLOODING, ... 174
" Causes of, ... 23
" Treatment of, ... 174
FRENCH SECRET, ... 144
" For what purpose used, . . . 144
" Its use in France,. 144
INTRODUCTORY REMARKS, ... ix
INFANTS, still born, ... 202
" Treatment of, ... 203
INFLAMMATION OF THE BREASTS, . . 205
" To prevent inflamed or broken Breasts, 208
Index, ... v
LABOUR—Signs of, ... 182
" Management of, ... 185
" Ordinary or natural, ... 186
Preternatural or Cross Births, . 201
Laborious, or difficult, ... 202
" Directions during, ... 198
" Directions after, . . . 99,203
MALFORMATION of the Pelvis, ... 180
MENSTRUATION, or Monthly Turns, ... 1
" RETENTION OF. 8
" Description, ... 8
" Causes, ... 8
" Symptoms, . . 9
" Treatment, ... 10
SUPPRESSION OF, ... 11
Description of, ... 11
Causes, ... 12
Symptoms, ... 12
Treatment of, ... 13
Specific certain to effect a cure, . 16
PAINFUL AND IMPERFECT, . . 18
Symptoms. 19
" Causes, ... 19
" Treatment, ... 20
MENSES—
" IMMODERATE FLOW OF, . . . 22
" Symptoms, ... 22
Causes, ... 23
Treatment, ... 23
Prevention, ... 27

		Page
MENSES—		
"	Decline of the,	28
"	Symptoms,	30
"	Causes,	30
"	Treatment,	33
MISCARRIAGE—*See Abortion.*		
MORAND'S "ELIXIR,"		232
"	Its success in effecting Cures,	233
NAVEL CORD—		
"	Manner of tying,	198
NURSING,		204
PORTUGUESE FEMALE PILLS,		16
PREFACE,		iii
PREGNANCY, Signs of,		36
"	How it may be determined,	37
"	Ceasing to be unwell,	38
	Morning Sickness,	49, 62
"	Shooting Pains through, Enlargement of and other Changes of the Breasts,	50
	Changes of the Nipple,	51
"	Presence of Milk,	54
"	Quickening,	57
PREGNANCY,—Diseases of,		61
"	Being unwell during,	96
"	Costiveness,	72
	Diarrhœa,	76
	Enlargement of the Veins of the Legs,	82
	Fainting Fits,	87
	Heart-Burn,	70
	Headache,	98
	Inconvenience from size,	95
	Painful and distended condition of the Breasts,	90
	Pains in the Legs, &c.,	92
	Palpitation of the Heart,	85
	Piles,	78
	Salivation, or Discharge of Saliva,	89
	Swelling of the Feet and Legs,	84
	Soreness and Cracking of the Skin of the Abdomen,	94
	Toothache,	88
	Violent movement of the Child,	93

		Page
PREGNANCY—Prevention of,		104
"	When unnecessary,	110
"	When indispensable,	107
	Practicability of,	141
	Morality of,	146
	Social importance of,	114
	Mode of prevention,	142,143,144
	Healthiness of,	145
	Reasons for prevention,	144
	Objections answered,	146
	Proofs of success,	150,152,154
"	Use of in France and other parts of	
"	Europe,	149
SEXUAL WEAKNESS,		
"	Symptoms,	157
"	Causes,	158
"	Treatment,	158
"	Regimen,	163
WOMB, falling down of the.		63

INTRODUCTORY REMARKS.

In introducing a subject of the nature treated of in this volume we are perhaps treading upon interdicted if not dangerous ground, for the world is not free from those pseudo-moralists, who would check, and, if possible, arrest the onward progress of medical and physiological science, and compel all to trudge on in the old beaten path, neither turning to the left nor the right, much less to look forward, but cast their glance backward. And although they behold every other science marching with rapid strides to comparative perfection :—what through the agency of steam and iron rails, space as it were, annihilated; what but yesterday, comparatively speaking, required weeks to perform, a few hours now suffice; nay the lightning fluid itself is made subservient to man's powers of dis covery and ingenuity, transmitting intelligence from distant points with the speed of thought :—yet, in physiological and medical science, we are required to be as an immovable rock, upon which the overwhelming billows of physiological science and discovery are to wash fruitlessly and in vain, to recede back into the dark sea of ignorance.

Truly, is it that in all that concerns man's welfare and woman's happiness, we are to stand still, while improvements and discoveries, in arts and sciences connected with agricultural and mechanical pursuits, are rushing by with the impetus of a torrent? Is it that physiological and medical science has long since reached that state of perfection that improvement and discovery are impossible? Is it that preceding generations had engrossed, in physiology, all the knowledge that could be attained, and left nothing for succeeding generations to attain? Is it that disease, decrepitude, bodily suffering and stinted and imperfect physical development among mankind has no longer an existence? Is it that every woman enjoys the full bloom, virgin freshness and beauty belonging to the enjoyment of a perfect condition of health? Is it that we no longer behold the deathly pale, sallow, sickly female of sixteen or eighteen, in the last stage of some chronic disease, prepared for the cold embrace of death? Is it that for the married woman six of the nine months of pregnancy is often a state of suffering and anguish destructive to her health and cutting off her days? Is it too, that it never happens that she often has children only at the hazard of her own life, and that of her offspring? Is it that children are invariably born healthy and rugged, capable of enduring the ordinary maladies to which infancy may be subject, to be reared into robust and virtuous sons and daughters? Is it that by far the greatest proportion of those born, survive, instead of, at the least, two-thirds being cut off in infancy? No, indeed, it is not because of all this. It is because prejudice or ignorance thinks that if men and women acquired the knowledge whereby to improve their condition as social moral beings, guard against disease, and preserve their health, that *perhaps*, it might lead to immorality and vice. This is ever the pretext to arrest the progress of physiological discovery.

Discoveries, then, so directly and intimately connected with the personal individual happiness of every man, woman, and child, are alone to see no progress; without being met at the threshold with the senseless and idle cry of "vice and immorality." Thus then, the sufferings, the pains, the anguish, which have existed five hundred years ago, are to be irremediable and endured in despite of any discoveries *by which they can be prevented.* We must do nothing to alleviate, or better still, to prevent, the sufferings of the wife, daughter, or mother, because it was not done five hundred years ago! Monstrously absurd as is this reasoning, yet it is of this kind which the discoveries introduced before the public in this work will be met.

But the subject is one which embraces our social joys and comforts, the endearments of home and the family fire-side, the health and well-being of wives, mothers, and daughters, and cannot be retarded by the cobwebs in its way, to stem its onward course. No female, either married, or about to be married—no wife about becoming a mother—no mother having a daughter—no father who desires to prolong the health, beauty, and vigor of his offspring—no husband who has his own happiness, or the happiness of the companion of his bosom at heart—no young man, even, having a regard to his future welfare, should be without this important little work. Here the wife, mother or daughter, can detect her own complaints, trace them to their causes, and apply the remedy. This is all important. For, how often does the young female (because of a supposed delicacy), suffer in health rather than impart her malady to another, and especially to a medical man; and thus, many diseases, which though trifling in their origin, and at first easily removed, become seated and confirmed in her constitution. How deplorable are the consequences arising either from neglect or ignorance in the treatment of females who are afflicted with a stoppage, irregularity, or entire suppression of the menses or monthly turns, from which spring a train of diseases, which it would, in this place, be useless to enumerate, but which make our wives and daughters sickly, and our offspring short-lived.

It is also important that the female should understand the cause which might occasion a stoppage of the menses to possess the information contained in this work, by which it can be ascertained whether it may not arise from pregnancy and thereby avoid that anxiety of mind arising from an uncertainty as to her real situation, alternately imagining the one or the other, as her inclinations or fears may tend.

During pregnancy, many a wife lives in almost perpetual bodily ailment and suffering, which ought and should be prevented, and would not in most cases exist if this work is perused. Here important truths and discoveries are revealed, which may be the means of saving many an affectionate wife and fond mother from a premature grave. How many females marry, who, in becoming pregnant, jeopardize their life, would learn, if they perused these pages, of the discovery by which *pregnancy can be prevented*, by means at once safe, simple, certain, and healthy, and thus many a victim would not fall a sacrifice to the Cæsarean operation.

In respect, too, when a woman is threatened with miscarriage or abortion it is important that the treatment, either to prevent it, or, when that is impracticable, to assist and expedite it, should be thoroughly understood, and its treatment made clear and simple, that no unnecessary alarm need be occasioned when it occurs.

So, too, in regard to the various diseases accompanying and belonging to pregnancy, every woman should know how to prevent the one and ameliorate the other.

And finally, the subject of unfruitfulness, sterility, or barrenness, is here presented in a manner, which, to some extent, demonstrates that in most cases it can be cured, yet how many are pining in childless loneliness, in utter despair of cure.

Such are some of the important topics treated of in these pages, so intimately connected with every woman's peace and happiness, with which every woman should be conversant, and yet how little informed are most females with what concerns themselves their children and their husbands so much.

MANAGEMENT

OF

FEMALE COMPLAINTS

MENSTRUATION.

One of the principal constitutional characteristics of the female, is menstruation, or the monthly evacuations peculiar to the sex.

This important operation generally takes place about the age of twelve or thirteen; but varies through the world, either in degree or frequency, both from constitution and climate.

Women in the higher ranks of life, and those of a delicate, nervous constitution, are subject to sickness, head-ache, and pains in the back and loins, during periodical evacuation. Those of the lower rank, inured to exercise and labor, and strangers to those refinements which debilitate the system, and interupt the functions essential to the preservation of health, are seldom observed to suffer at these times, unless from general indisposition, or a diseased state of the womb.

After the discharge has become established it recurs periodically while in health; and its recurrence is so regular, that it can be calculated with great exactness. The usual period of its visitations is from twenty-seven to thirty days. As to the time of its continuance, this is various in different women; but it seldom continues longer than six days, or less than three, and does not cease suddenly but in a gradual manner.

Its approach is generally preceded by certain feelings of oppression or deviation from the ordinary state of health, which warn the individual of what is to happen. There is, in particular, a sensation of fulness about the lower part of the belly, and a relaxation about the uterine system which can scarcely be overlooked by the most heedless. The appetite becomes delicate, the limbs tremble and feel weak, the face becomes pale, and there is a peculiar dark streak or shade under the eyes; sometimes great restlessness, slight fever, head-ache, heavy and dull pain in the small of the back and bottom of the belly, swelled and hardened breasts, &c. All of which are sometimes instantly relieved by a trifling discharge from the vagina, and this not necessarily colored. It must at the same time be admitted, that in some few constitutions these feelings are so inconsiderable as to be little attended to; so that the woman mixes in society as usual without any apparent inconvenience.

The period at which the menses make their appearance, is various; it is much influenced by constitution, climate and mode of life. As a general rule, it takes place at puberty, or at that period at which the female is capable of propagating her species; and this period varies as climate may differ. They constantly, however, keep pace with the development of the body; where this is rapid, they will appear proportionably earlier; where this process is slower, they will appear later; but whenever the menses appear as regular evacuations, they mark the period of puberty: thus, in hot countries, women commence to menstruate at eight or nine years of age, and are not unfrequently mothers at ten.*

In the more northern regions, as in Lapland, &c., this evacuation is generally delayed until the female has attained her eighteenth or nineteenth yéar: in the temperate latitudes the average period will be found from the fourteenth to the sixteenth year. A difference, will, nevertheless, be found in the women who may reside in cities, and in

* The following table exhibits the ages of three hundred and twenty-six females, at which they began to menstruate. It is furnished me by Mr. Robertson, in the *North of England Medical and Surgical Journal.*

In their 11th year,	6	In their 16th year,	54
12th "	12	17th "	50
13th "	31	18th "	19
14th "	60	19th "	18
15th "	72	20th "	4

To this list may be added the case related by Madame Boivin, in her account of a new case of abortion. The subject of this case commenced to menstruate at seven years of age, and did so regularly after her tenth year those who dwell in the country of each respective portion of the globe. It may also be observed, that in cold countries, women continue to menstruate for a longer period than in warm; and as a general rule, it will be found they are obnoxious to this discharge double the period that elapses before it commences. Thus, women who have not this discharge until eighteen, will be found to have it until beyond fifty; those who commence at fourteen or fifteen, will leave off at forty-five; those who begin so early as eight or nine, will have it cease at twenty-five or six.*

On the appearance of the menses, or monthly turns, nature seems to perfect her work, both as regards development and proportion: it is the period of the most perfect beauty of which the female is susceptible; it is the one at which the moral changes are not less remarkable than the physical; it is a moment, of all others, the most replete with consequences to the inexperienced and confiding female.

* We could record a number of instances where the menses were continued much beyond their ordinary period, and where, after ceasing some time, they were resumed with their accustomed regularity; but we shall limit our observations to one case, and that because it is recent and well authenticated This case is recorded in the *Ann. Univ. de Med.* A female aged ninety-four continued to menstruate from the fifty-third to the ninety-fourth year. Her relatives were remarkable for their longevity; she is at present in perfect health.—*American Journal of the Medical Sciences for Feb.* 1831

At this period a great variety of interesting and curious phenomena present themselves: the voice is found to change; the neck and throat to increase in size, and to become more symmetrical; the mammæ to swell; the nipple to protrude; the chest to expand; the eyes to acquire intelligence, and increase of brilliancy; in a word, a new being, almost, is created.

The quantity of fluid expended at a menstruous period differs in different individuals; with girls who precociously menstruate, the quantity is in general smaller, and the returns less regular. Climate exerts an influence upon the quantity discharged, as well as upon the periods at which this evacuation shall commence. Thus, in the equatorial and more northern regions, it is less than in the more temperate climates.

It is of importance for women to know that occasional irregularities are not always the consequences of disease. Constitutions vary as much in respect to the regular returns of this discharge, as they do with regard to their first appearance or final cessation. Those in whom the change occurs very early from vigor of constitution, require little to be done for them; but in weak and delicate habits, the non-appearance of this evacuation is too often considered as the cause, whereas it ought to be viewed as the effect, of the state of the habit unpropitious to its taking place. And, according to family practice, under this false impression, warm teas and forcing medicines are employed at the approach of this disease, which have often done much harm.

Nature is not so defective in her own udgment as to require auxiliaries. Car bould be taken to improve the general state of the health, by attention to diet, moderate exercise, change of air, &c.

In some instances the menstrual discharge does not make its appearance before the age of seventeen or eighteen, and, neverthe-less, health is not in the least affected. The mere want of evacuation at the ordinary time, therefore, is not to be considered as morbid, unless the system be evidently de-ranged thereby. In many cases, however, symptoms of disease appear which are evi-dently connected with the defect of the menses, and go off upon its discharge. The treatment, in such cases, must be regulated by the particular circumstances and consti-tution of the individual. There is no remedy adapted to every case of this kind; but an open state of the bowels, and a due regula tion of the diet, together with moderate ex-ercise, are useful in every instance of this omplaint. Warm clothing, too, particularly bout the lower extremities, is of mos essential benefit. The occasional use of the warm bath is pleasant and beneficial, espe-cially if the skin be dry and warm. As the health improves, the cold bath will prove an auxiliary, if, after using it, the patient feels a glow of heat and a greater degree of liveliness. When the means ordinarily employed have failed, marriage, or a change of climate, has produced the wished-for effect.

In some instances the evacuation is impeded by a mechanical cause, that is an obstruction of the passage to the womb. This occasionally is met with, and the chief obstacle to its speedy removal is the difficulty of ascertaining its existence. The operation by which it is completely remedied, is not more painful nor formidable than blood-letting.

Fortunately, in most cases, the evacuation takes place in due time, and the constitution sustains no material or permanent injury. It is, however, in every instance, proper to pay particular attention to the system during the continuance of the evacuation.

The stomach and bowels, at this period, are very easily disordered, and therefore, everything which is heavy or indigestible, ought to be avoided. Some are hurt by eating fruits or vegetables; others by taking fermented liquor. In this respect experience must enable each individual to judge for herself. Exposure to cold, particularly getting the feet wet, is hurtful, as it tends suddenly to obstruct the discharge. The same effec is likewise produced by violent passions of the mind, which are also, at this time, peculiarly apt to excite spasmodic affections, or hysterical fits.

It is, in general, a very proper rule not to administer any very active medicines, at this time, unless some violent symptom absolutely requires them. Opiates, for instance, are, in many cases, necessary to allay spasmodic affections, or abate pain; and they are, in such circumstances, uniformly safe. They give speedy relief to hysterical feeling or suffocation, or to spasm of the stomach or bowels.

Dancing, exposure to much heat, or making any great or fatiguing exertion, are improper. These causes may increase, to an improper degree, the quantity of the evacuation, and in certain circumstances may give a disposition to a falling down of the womb

---

RETENTION OF THE MENSES.

Description.

The menstrual discharge is liable, from many causes, to become obstructed at the period when it ought to appear; when this takes place it is attended with very painful or serious effects; and, if nature is not assisted, the health is impaired or the constitution undermined, inducing consumption or some other complaint.

Causes.

The remote cause of this complaint is mos

frequently suppressed perspiration; and it may arise, in part, from an inactive sedentary life, and such habits as are peculiar to the higher classes of society, particularly in cities and towns. The proximate cause of it seems to be a want of power in the system, arising from inability to propel the blood into the uterine vessels with sufficient force to open their extremities and to allow a discharge of blood from them.

Symptoms.

Heaviness, listlessness to motion, fatigue on the least exercise, palpitation of the heart, pains in the back, loins, and hips, flatulence, acidities in the stomach and bowels, costiveness, a perternatural appetite for chalk, lime, and various other absorbents, together with many other dyspeptic symptoms. As it advances in its progress the face becomes pale, and afterward assumes a yellowish hue, even verging upon green, whence it has been called green sickness; the lips lose their rosy color; the eyes are encircled with a livid areola; the whole body has an unhealthy appearance, with every indication of a want of power and energy in the constitution; the feet are affected with swellings; the breathing is much hurried by any great exertion of the body; the pulse is quick, but small; and the person is liable to a cough, and to many of the symptoms of hysteria. Sometimes a great quantity of pale urine is discharged in the morning, and not unfrequently hectic fever attends. In cases of a more chronic character there is a continued, though variable, state of sallowness, yellowness, darkness, or a wan, squalid, or sordid paleness of complexion, or ring of darkness surrounding the eyes, and extending perhaps a little toward the temples and cheeks.

Treatment.

As this disease proceeds from debility, it is evident that the great object to be fulfilled will be to give tone and energy to the system; and if this debility has arisen from a sedentary life, the patient must begin immediately to exercise in the open air, and, if practicable, to change her residence. The tepid or warm bath should be used in preference to the cold. The first medicine given may be the pulverized *mandrake root*, combined with a little *cream of tartar*. This, as well as other medicines, should be taken upon an empty stomach: after it has been given, *motherwort*, *pennyroyal*, and other herb teas may be freely drunk. After the exhibition of the purgative, which may be occasionally repeated, *gum aloes* may be taken, combined in such a manner as to prevent the piles. This medicine, from its action upon the uterus through the medium of the rectum, is very useful in retention of the menses. *Emmenagogues*, or "forcing medicines," should not be used to bring on the menses, except there be a struggle or effort of nature to effect it, which may be known by the periodical pains and pressing down about the hips and loins. When this occurs let the feet be bathed, and perspiration promoted, by drinking freely of diluent teas, such as *pennyroyal*, *motherwort*, and *garden thyme*. Should considerable pains attend the complaint, eight or ten grains of the *diaphoretic powders* may be given, and *fomentations of bitter herbs* applied over the region of the womb. *Desomeaux's Portuguese Pills* are now recommended as the best specific, especially if the disease proves obstinate.

The female should be very careful not to expose herself to the vicissitudes of the weather, and not suffer the feet or clothes to become wet: warm clothing must be worn, and particularly flannel. For pain apply a heated brick, covered, to the bowels.

The diet should be light, nutritious, and easy of digestion.

SUPPRESSION OF THE MENSES.

Description.

In this disease there is a partial or total obstruction of the menses in women from other causes than pregnancy and old age

The menses should be regular as to the quantity and quality; that this discharge should observe the monthly period, is essential to health. When it is obstructed, nature makes her efforts to obtain for it some other outlet; if these efforts of nature fail, the consequence may be, fever, pulmonic diseases, spasmodic affections, hysteria, epilepsy, mania, apoplexy, green sickness, according to the general habit and disposition of the patient. Any interruption occurring after the menses have once been established in their regular course, except when occasioned by conception, is always to be considered as a case of suppression. A constriction of the extreme vessels, arising from accidental events, such as cold, anxiety of mind, fear, inactivity of body, irregularities of diet. putting on damp clothes, the frequent use of acids and other sedatives, &c., is the cause which evidently produces a suppression of the menses. This shows the necessity for certain cautions and attentions during the discharge. In some few cases it appears as a symptom of other diseases, and particularly of general debility in the system, showing a want of due action of the vessels. When the menses have been suppressed for any considerable length of time, it not unfrequently happens that the blood which should have passed off by the uterus, being determined more copiously and forcibly to other parts, gives rise to hemorrhages; hence it is frequently poured out from the nose, stomach lungs, and other parts, in such cases. At first, however, febrile or inflammatory symptoms appear, the pulse is hard and frequent, the skin hot, and there is a severe pain in the head, back, and loins. Besides, the patient is likewise much troubled with costiveness, colic pains, and dyspeptic and hysteric symptoms.

Treatment.

It will be necessary, in the treatment of this disease, to remove urgent symptoms if they are present. If the patient is in severe pain, give the *diaphoretic powders*,* and at the same time let a strong infusion of *garden thyme* and *pennyroyal* be freely given. Im-

* *Diaphoretic Powder.*

Take of Gum Opium, - - - -	half a drachm
Camphor, - - - -	two drachms
Pulverized Ipecacuanha, -	one drachm
Cream of Tartar, or super-carbonate of soda, - - -	one ounce

Pulverize all separately, then mix. It is best to use pulverized opium.

Dose—Ten grains, or half a tea-spoonful, as often as may be necessary.

Use—This forms a valuable anodyne, diaphoretic and sudorific. It is beneficially administered in fever, St. Anthony's fire, diarrhœa, dysentery, and cholera morbus, and in all cases where an anodyne, combined with a sudorific, is required. In these diseases it should be administered in small doses. It is also applicable to many other diseases, such as rheumatism, gout, &c. It promotes perspiration without increasing the heat of the body. It produces a constant moisture of the skin for a great length of time, while it allays irritation.

merse the feet in warm lye water, and rub well with coarse flannel. If relief is not obtained in the course of an hour, or in a very short time, a strong decoction of bitter herbs should be thrown into a proper vessel and the patient steamed fifteen or twenty times, as long as she is able to bear, or until perspiration is produced; immediately after which let her be put in bed, covered warm, and the herbs be enclosed in flannel or muslin, and applied to the lower part of the abdomen or belly. This process will almost immediately relieve the urgent symptoms. After this our next object will be, to regulate the menstrual discharge, by a proper course of strengthening medicine; that recommended under the head of *chlorosis*, or *a retention of the menses*, may be taken with advantage. Inasmuch as both proceed from debility, it is evident that it must be removed in order to effect a cure; and, therefore, that medicine and treatment which strengthen and invigorate the system, will invariably benefit the patient. The skin, stomach, and intestines, all seem concerned in the production of this disease, and hence our attention should be directed to a restoration of their proper offices: the stomach and bowels should be cleansed and stimulated to a healthy action; perspiration must be promoted, and, in short, every secretion and excretion of the system. If the stomach is in a morbid condition, let an emetic be occasionally given, and afterwards a dose of *mandrake;* both of which may be repeated as occasion requires. The patient may then take the following tonic bitters: Take prickly ash bark, two ounces; wild cherry tree bark, two ounces; Seneca snake-root, one ounce; tanzy, one ounce; gum socotrine aloes, half an ounce; devil's bit, two ounces: pulverize; to every two ounces of the powder add half a pint of boiling water and one quart of Holland gin, and half a wine-glassful taken three or four times a day. This may be continued while it agrees with the patient, or as long as benefit is derived. About once a month there will generally be felt more or less symptoms preceding a catamenial discharge; considerable pain will be felt through the lower part of the abdomen, hips, and loins, showing that there is a strong effort or struggle of nature to return the menses. Our principal object, when this occurs, should be, to aid her salutary efforts, as directed in the Retention of the Menses. The patient should sit over the steam of *bitter herbs* for ten or fifteen minutes, retaining the steam by means of a blanket, to concentrate it upon the lower part of the body; at the same time the feet may be bathed, and tansy tea freely drunk. The abdomen should also be fomented, as before directed. It will not be necessary, however, to use these means, except there is an obvious indication to return the menses.*

* The most successful specific, and one almost invariably

It must be recollected that when the patient labors under some other disease, there

certain in removing a stoppage, irregularity, or suppression of the menses (monthly turn), is a compound invented by M. M. Desomeaux, of Lisbon, Portugal, called the Portuguese Female Pills. It would appear that they are infallible, and would, undoubtedly, even produce miscarriage, if exhibited during pregnancy. And what is equally important, they are always mild, healthy, and safe in their effects.

In the female hospitals in Vienna and Paris, their exhibition has entirely superseded the use of the ordinary remedies; because, where a cure is attainable by medicinal remedies, they are certain of success. Their astonishing efficacy would be almost incredible, if not vouched for by indubitable testimony, in numerous instances producing returns of the monthly periods after all hope had been abandoned. A remarkable case is related by Dr. A. M. Mauriceau, during his residence in Paris.

"While residing in Paris, I had frequent opportunities of witnessing the astonishing efficacy of the Portuguese Female Pills in obstinate cases of the suppression of the menses. Their effect, in one instance in particular, seemed almost miraculous. A young lady, about twenty years of age, of wealthy and respectable parentage, had not menstruated for nearly two years before her application to me. On inquiry, I ascertained that her health was not seriously affected (except at intervals of about four weeks, occasioned, doubtless, by the efforts of nature to perform her functions), until within the preceding four months, when her symptoms began to assume an alarming appearance. Her medical attendants here prescribed the usual remedies without success.

"I must confess, I thought her case desperate, and had but little hope that Desomeaux's celebrated Portuguese Pills, which I determined to put to the test, would here avail, as I had never known them to be administered under circumstances quite so apparently hopeless for a cure. But I resolved upon a trial. Accordingly I recommended their use, watching their effects upon the patient. At first their virtue, so to speak, seemed is such debility that there is not superfluous blood sufficient to keep up the menstrual discharge; and in this case our attention must

to be only negative—that is, the young woman got no worse. This, however, under the circumstances, I considered a point gained. In the course of three weeks favorable indications began to present themselves. The appetite was better; the deathly-sallow complexion giving place to a healthy hue; the eyes, also, becoming clearer, but still no menstrual discharge. The improvement, however, meanwhile, became more and more apparent, till, at the end of the ninth week after commencing their use, a slight, somewhat reddish discharge took place. Here was a beginning; the patient still improving, taking moderate exercise, with light but nourishing diet. Their exhibition was then dispensed with until within five or six days just previous to the expected return of the menses, when they were again used, and their use continued during the seven days; on the eighth the menses again appeared—on this occasion somewhat freer, but still not in sufficient quantity Their exhibition ceased with the cessation of the menses, which lasted irregularly about four days. This treatment continued to the end of the fourth month, when the monthly returns were perfectly established. At each successive appearance they assumed a healthier color, freer in quantity, and less obstructed by coagula. The patient entirely recovered, and became possessed of sound health."

He then relates another instance still more surprising. "A woman applied to be treated for suppression. It appeared that she had been subject to irregularity, or stoppage of the monthly turns, and as she appeared to be free from the usual symptoms attending pregnancy, it was not supposed that the stoppage arose from tha cause. She commenced using Desomeaux's Pills. After using them about five days—from certain indications attending miscarriage—apprehensions began to be entertained that the suppression might have arisen from pregnancy, which, upon examination, proved to be the case —too late, however, to prevent the miscarriage. In a short time the expulsion took place, and on about the be directed to the primary affection, without any regard to such symptoms ; it is also very necessary to bear in mind the fact, that the menses are often suppressed from pregnancy. By a proper attention, we can always discriminate between a suppression of the menses and pregnancy ; and the principal diagnostic symptom is, that in the former complaint there is a pain or affection of the head, attended with dizziness.

PAINFUL AND IMPERFECT MENSTRUATION.

Description.

Besides the two deviations from the usual

course of nature already mentioned, there sometimes occurs a third, viz. where menstruation, although not wholly suppressed, is nevertheless somewhat difficult, and accompanied with severe pains in the back, loins and bottom of the belly. This disease is owing to a weak action of the vessels of the uterus, or spasm of its extreme vessels, and is to be obviated by tonics, warm bathing, both local and general, together with the use of anodynes, which should be employed as soon as the symptoms which denote its approach are apparent. This complaint is a common, and generally an extremely harassing, affection. It may occur at every period during the menstruation stage of life; but it appears to be most common between the twentieth and thirtieth years of age, and in subjects of an irritable and sanguineous temperament. In many instances severe pains are experienced in the back, loins, and lower part of the abdomen for five or six hours previous to the appearance of the menses. This, however, soon ceases, and an immediate aggravation of the torturing pain follows. Sometimes the catamenia begin to flow moderately, with little or no previous pains; but in an hour or two, they become suddenly arrested, at the same time that violent pains come on in the hips, side, loins, back, and thighs, with a distressing sensation of forcing or bearing down. Occasionally a very slight menstrual discharge continues uninterruptedly for three or four days, accompanied throughout with extremely severe pains in the abdomen; and in some rare instances the catamenial evacuation, although attended with great suffering, is sufficiently copious and prolonged in its course, and may even exceed the regular duration and quantity of an ordinary healthy menstruation.

Treatment.

Since it is well known that a derangement in the uterine functions must generally proceed from a check of perspiration, astringing the minute ends of the uterine vessels, or in some manner deranging their functions, causing debility, &c., it will appear clear that our first attention must be directed to the skin. Cold appears to be the cause of the disease, and heat seems to remove it; therefore, when these periods of distress occur, let the patient sit over a strong decoction of bitter herbs, such as tansy, hoarhound, wormwood, catnip and hops, while a blanket is thrown round the waist of the patient to confine the steam to the lower parts. After the diseased person has been thus steamed and the feet bathed, let her be put into a bed, warmly covered, and diluent drinks given, such as tansy, thyme, pennyroyal, &c. At the same time let fomentations of the same herbs, enclosed in a flannel bag, be applied to the abdomen, as before directed. This will produce perspiration and afford immediate relief; and when these distressing symptoms are removed, and the patient becomes comfortable, a course of treatment must be adopted to prevent a recurrence of these symptoms, or to produce a natural flow of the catamenial discharge; and similar to that recommended under the preceding complaints. Herbs may be freely drunk.

A writer on this subject thus remarks. "This case of painful menstruation deserves particular attention, because it impairs the health of patients by its present effects, and seems to render them less prolific in future. Dr. Fothergill has afforded relief to several by the following process: Let the patient have near her a few pills, consisting of opium gr. i. each, made soft with a little of any kind of conserve. She is to take one of these pills the moment the pain attending this discharge comes on. A pill may be taken every hour till the pain ceases: more than two will seldom be required; yet they must be taken in quantities sufficient to mitigate the pain. Let the patient keep either in or upon the bed, or at least in a recumbent posture, drink moderately of any diluting liquor, as herb teas, weak whey, or thin broth. When the time is past, a course of chalybeate bitters, in small doses, may be continued, till within a few days of the return; and the bowels should be kept open with some proper laxative. This excruciating pain seems to be spasmodic, and to proceed from the extreme irritability of the uterine system." The *diaphoretic powders* will be found very useful. Diet and exercise are important. A hot brick or salt, enclosed in flannel wet with vinegar, and applied to the bowels, soon relieves the pain

---

IMMODERATE FLOW OF THE MENSES.

This alarming complaint may occur under two different states of the constitution. In the one, the woman is of full habit, and often of a ruddy countenance. In the other, she is pale, delicate, and easily fatigued.

Symptoms.

In plethoric habits it is often preceded by head-ache, giddiness, or difficult breathing, and is afterwards attended with pain in the back and loins, universal heat, and a frequent, strong, and hard pulse. But when it arises from general debility, or in consequence of a laxity of the organ, paleness of the face, chilliness, lassitude of the body, oppressed breathing on the slightest effort, pains in the back on remaining any length of time in an erect posture, and coldness of the extremities, together with a long train of nervous complaints.

Causes.

A variety of causes may produce this troublesome disease. Some of these are general, such as a state of great weakness, or of too much blood; others are local, such as debility of the uterus, occasioned by tedious labor or frequent miscarriages. It may also be produced by accidental circumstances determining the blood more copiously and forcibly into the uterine vessels, as violent exercise in dancing, much straining at stool from great costiveness, contusion on the belly, excess in venery, or strong passions of the mind, particularly at the menstrual period.

Treatment.

In the management of this disease we have two objects: first, to moderate the discharge and procure present security; and, secondly, to prevent a return.

The first thing to be done when the hemorrhage is sudden or profuse, is instantly to remove the clothing which may occasion the least interruption to the free circulation of the blood, and to put the patient to bed, lightly covered with clothes. So long as this discharge continues, it is of importance to keep her in a recumbent posture, as cool as possible, and perfectly at rest, both in body and mind. Cloths, dipped in cold vinegar and water, and renewed as often as they become warm. These cold applications have a powerful effect in restraining uterine hemorrhage, and ought never to be omitted where the discharge of blood is profuse.

If the patient be of a full habit, attended with severe pain in the head or back, and febrile symptoms, it will be proper to give the antimonial, or febrifuge powders, or mixture.*

The state of the belly must be attended to. It can be kept gently open by the cathartic mixture, sulphur, or any mild laxative medicine. Stimulating purgatives or clysters, under such circumstances, are improper, from their tendency to increase the discharge.

When no symptoms indicating an increased action in the vessels of the womb are present, astringent medicines should be employed. And, in cases where the discharges have not continued long, and the strength not much impaired, it is often sufficient to

* *Antimonial Powders.*—Take of tartar emetic, three grains, nitre, two drachms. Mix, and divide into two doses. One dose to be taken every two or three hours by adults. In obstinate cases, the addition of ten or twelve grains of calomel to the above recipe, will render the medicine more salutary.

Febrifuge Powders.—Take of ipecacuanha, two scruples; nitre, two drachms.—Mix, and divide into twelve doses. One dose to be taken every two or three hours by adults.

Febrifuge Mixture.—Take of nitre, two drachms; lemon juice or vinegar, one ounce; water, half a pint, sugar, a sufficient quantity to sweeten.—Mix. A wine-glassful to be taken by adults every two hours. It will be rendered more active by the addition of two drachms of antimonial wine arrest the disease by giving fifteen or twenty drops of elixir vitriol, or six or eight grains of alum dissolved in a glass of cold water every hour; or, what is preferable, alum whey, sweetened to the taste, in doses of a small cupful, as often as the stomach will receive it. But, if the discharge be obstinate, we should have recourse to pills of sugar of lead and opium.*

In no instance which has come under my knowledge, where the hemorrhage was in consequence of a laxity of the uterine vessels, have these pills failed in producing the desired effect.

In those cases where the hemorrhage is profuse, or of long continuance, and resists the means already pointed out, it will be proper to inject into the uterus from a gill to half a pint of a strong decoction of oak bark, in which one or two drachms of alûm have been dissolved, or as much of the saturated solution of alum in water, in order to constringe and strengthen the vessels of the womb. This may be repeated twice or thrice a day, according to circumstances.

When symptoms of an increased action in the vessels of the womb are observable, the

* *Pills of Sugar of Lead.*—Take of sugar of lead and ipecacuanha, each six grains; opium, one grain; syrup sufficient to form a mass.—Divide in four parts; one part to be taken every three hours, until the hemorrhage ceases; or pulv. opii, four gr.; pulv. sugar of lead. twelve grs. Mix, and divide in four parts; give one in a little water, in an hour give half of another

tincture of foxglove, in doses of twenty drops every four hours, constitutes the best remedy.

When there is reason to suppose the hemorrhage proceeds from a scirrhous or ulcerated state of the womb, all that can be done is to afford temporary relief by giving opium in large doses. Indeed, opiates may be given with advantage in every case where there is considerable pain or anxiety, and the patient much exhausted. Under these circumstances, from one to two teaspoonfuls of laudanum, or from two to four grains of opium, according to the urgency of the case, will be useful not only in giving a check to the discharge, but also in preserving the strength, and abating nervous irritation. In most cases it is preferable to give opium in the form of injections to allay the spasmodic pains of the womb; and, when administered in this way, clysters of thin starch or gruel, in each of which two teaspoonfuls of laudanum are added, should be given every two hours until relief be obtained. (*See Abortion and Flooding.*)

Regimen.

The diet, at the time of excessive discharge, must be light and cool. The drink must always be cold, as ice-water, lemonade, or tamarind beverage. Port wine, in such cases, is too frequently resorted to, which uniformly does harm by increasing the circulation.

Prevention.

To prevent a recurrence of the attack in those who are subject to it, the patient must necessarily avoid the causes by which it has been produced.

When it is evident that the discharge is in consequence of a full habit, it will be proper to reduce the system by living sparingly, by keeping the bowels rather in a laxative state, and by rising early, and taking through the day regular but frequent exercise ; and, after the plethora is removed, by strengthening the vessels which have been over-distended, by the use of the cold bath.

In a greater number of cases, however, we meet with a delicate constitution and spare habit, with pale countenance : this state requires the use of sea bathing or the shower bath, and the vessels of the womb are particularly strengthened by pouring cold water daily on the back and loins.

It will be advisable to use a generous nutritive diet, with wine, and to have recourse to some of the tonic medicines, as advised under the head of obstructed menses, to strengthen the system generally. At the same time the bowels must be attended to, and invigorating exercise taken daily ; whilst on the other hand, fatigue, and especially exposure to relaxing heat, must be carefully avoided.

DECLINE OF THE MENSES.

The nearer a woman approaches her forty-fifth year (*cæteris paribus*), will be the risk of some irregularity in the menses; and as this period is more frequently the one at which any latent disease of the uterus shows itself, it is always looked forward to with much anxiety by women. Indeed, so replete is this time with horrors to many, that we may very justly suspect apprehension to be the cause of some of the distressing symptoms, which sometimes accompany this interesting process of the human uterus.

Delicate women, and especially those who have lived idly, have this period of life arrive earlier than those of a contrary constitution, and opposite habits. We have already noticed, in our section on Suppression that this change sometimes takes place at a very early period of life, and this without leaving any injurious consequences behind it; and, on the other hand, we find many cases on record, where this discharge had continued with regularity to a much longer period than the ordinary one. Gardien mentions a case which fell under his own notice, where this evacuation continued with great exactness, until beyond the seventy-fifth year; others, still more uncommon, are mentioned by various writers.*

This change is sometimes effected so silently, that the woman scarcely notices her altered condition; at others, its approach is so gradual, as not to attract observation, until the diminished quantity gives warning that it is about to take its leave for ever; while, again, the irregularity, both in period and quantity, may be such, as justly to give alarm, as well as to produce the most serious danger.

But, as a general rule, it may be observed, that when the woman arrives at about her forty-fifth year, she finds her menses to become irregular, both in the quantity of fluid evacuated, and in the periods they observe; being sometimes in advance, and at others, not appearing until long after the accustomed time. The woman also finds some alteration has taken place in her general health; she becomes pale, debilitated, and nervous; arising, however, for the most part, from the too frequent returns of this discharge, or its too great abundance.

At this time, also, the woman sometimes

* I have had, very lately, a lady under my care, who menstruates with the most perfect regularity; though she had labored under a prolapsus of the uterus to a great extent for several years. She is now in her sixty-fifth year. Her uterus is now effectually supported by a pessary, which has much improved her general health.—*Dewees*

becomes the victim of a strange illusion, should the menses not have returned for several periods; for she now supposes herself to be pregnant, as her abdomen enlarges, as do the mammæ; her appetite becomes capricious, or she has strange longings, &c., the whole of the rational signs of this condition being present, in her imagination, even to the motion of the child. This delusion is most common to women who marry late in life, and who are very desirous of offspring. Now the breasts lose their intumescency; the morning sickness vanishes; the swelling of the abdomen subsides; the imagined stirrings of the fœtus cease, or the sensation becomes so unequivocal as to satisfy that it arises from the movement of wind; and, to put everything beyond hope, the menses return in overwhelming quantity. It is highly proper, that practitioners, and especially the younger part of them, should be put upon their guard in respect to this condition of the patient, and not too easily yield credence to all her wishes may dictate, or absolutely to treat as an impossibility, a circumstance of which there is occasionally an example.

It seems that the apprehensions of this period of life have arisen mainly from the notions entertained of the final cause of the menses; namely, that it gives vent to peccant humours. But females should be made to know, that all this is purely the theory of the vulgar; as the menstrual blood is formed from the general mass; and, consequently if that be pure, the other will be; therefore the idea is altogether ill-founded. But unfortunately, whenever this discharge is less abundant than usual, the most serious fears are entertained, that there will be a retention of a portion, which will cause disease, either in the uterus itself, or in some other part of the body; hence, a diminished menstruous secretion is always more alarming to the female, than an unusual flow. But it may be well to remark, that there is a great difference between the cessation of this discharge, and the suppression of it. In the one instance, it is an event which nature has designed should take place, and is effected altogether by arrangements of the system itself; and, of course, one of its natural processes: in a word, as much so as its commencement; but the suppression, from some morbid agency, is in direct opposition to the intentions of nature, and will, of course, be followed by some baleful consequence, if it continue beyond a certain period.

The vulgar error, that "women at this period of life are always in danger," is replete with mischief to the suffering sex; and I feel it a duty to declare, that they are not necessarily more obnoxious to disease at this, than at any other period of their existence.*

* Indeed, it would seem that this period of female life is freer from diseases causing death, than almost any

That they are sometimes liable to a disease at this time; and that disease one of the most terrible in the long list of human infirmities, I admit; but must, nevertheless, insist that *Cancer* (the disease to which I allude, and the one so much dreaded) is more rare in the uterus than in certain other portions of the body; for instance, the mammæ; and, perhaps, I am within the truth, when I say, that there are three instances of the latter for one of the former If latent dispositions to disease, either in the uterus or other parts, become active about this period of life, it is not because the declining menses excite them; but because the disease is slow in developing itself, and is, perhaps, kept in check for a long time, by the menstrual discharge serving as an important evacuation; especially when the uterus may be the seat of the complaint. In such instances, the foundation of the disease was laid, perhaps, at the time when the menses were the most perfect, as regards period and quantity; consequently, they could have had no agency in its production; but, on the contrary, from its frequently relieving the en-

other. By some late observations made on the bills o mortality in France, by M. Boiniston of Chateauneuf, it appears that fewer women die between the ages of forty and fifty, than men, or indeed at any other period of their lives, after puberty. And, further, that if this change is effected without much disturbance, that they live not only longer than men, but are free from morbid inconveniences.

gorgement of the vessels, served to keep it in subjection for a long time; not as a specific discharge, but as a mere depletion; or, in other words, that if an equal quantity of blood could have been by any other means as certainly abstracted from the uterus, the same favorable result would have followed. Coincidences in the human system are so common, that they are frequently mistaken for cause and effect; hence the cessation of the menstrual discharge, and the appearance of scirrhi and cancers, are considered as cause and effect.

At this period of life, nothing will so effectually secure the woman against injuries which may arise from the irregularities of the menstrual discharge, as a well-regulated regimen. By regimen, in this place, we would wish to be understood, not only eating and drinking, but exercise of both body and mind, including the proper government of the passions; in a word, everything which relates to both moral and physical existence.

A well-ordered course of exercise in the open air in well-selected weather, and great simplicity of diet, is of the utmost importance to the female at this period of life, and should never be neglected, if it be possible to indulge in them. By these means, the nervous, muscular, vascular, and lymphatic systems are all preserved more certainly in equilibrium with each other, since they are the best calculated to ensure a reciprocation of their respective offices; and, consequently, to maintain that condition of the system, termed health. Hence, the justness of the remark, that the women who live in the country, and who exercise freely in the open air; who have fulfilled their duties scrupulously as mothers, by suckling their children, agreeably to the views of nature; who do not goad their systems by over-stimulating food and drinks; who do not relax their bodies by too long indulgence in bed, have but little suffering at this period.

From this it will follow, that a milk and vegetable diet, together with pure water as a drink; regular exercise, not carried to fatigue; keeping the bowels well open, by well-selected food, as the fruits of the season in proper quantities: the bran bread if necessary; but not by medicine, unless absolutely required; governing the temper; restraining the passions, as well mental as animal, will largely contribute to the safety and comfort of this period. All that we have just recommended, is calculated to place the system in a condition by which it shall preserve its various forces; have its irritability diminished; its sensibility moderated; and pretty certainly prevent that condition of the blood-vessels, most decidedly unfriendly to the general health at this time, called plethora. And, though last, not least in fair estimation, is an attention to cleanliness. The external organs should be washed with lukewarm water at least twice a day, and the whole body once a week, by going into a lukewarm bath. In using the bath, care should be taken to come out of it as soon as the purposes of cleanliness are answered.

Our next concern is with the derangement of the discharge at or about the period of cessation: this will consist, 1st, in a diminution of the proper quantity; and, 2dly, in an excess of it. As regards the first, we have already said enough when treating of the suppression of the menses; and, with respect to the second, it must be treated according to the rules prescribed for the management of hemorrhage from the uterus from any other cause, that is, first, to diminish the quantity discharging; secondly, to prevent an excessive return

CONCEPTION;

OR,

PREGNANCY.

CONCEPTION.

In order to procreate the human species, there is a periodical discharge of blood from the vagina of every female, termed the catamenia, or menses. The secretion of this fluid commences at that period of life termed puberty, which occurs at different ages, according to the climate. In some latitudes it commences as early as eight or ten, and in others not until fifteen. As soon as conception or pregnancy commences, this discharge ceases, and goes to support the fœtus, or the child.

The manner in which conception takes place has ever been a fruitful subject of in quiry, but we are unable to account for thi change precisely. It is, however, pretty evident that the semen of the male is introduced into the uterus, while the semen of the female is discharged from the ovaria by means of the Fallopian tubes, the fimbricated extremity of which closely embraces that organ.

These tubes, by a kind of peristaltic motion similar to the intestines, convey the semen of the female into the uterus, where it unites with the semen of the male; and it is these united fluids which constitute the rudiment of the fœtus, and which often give to the child the appearance and dispositions of their parents. Sometimes one trait is inherited, sometimes another; at other times a new compound or character is formed (like a chemical union), which does not partake of the nature of either of the former.

OF THE MODE BY WHICH PREGNANCY MAY BE DETERMINED.

There are certain signs which a female is taught to regard as essential evidences of pregnancy; and it is supposed by most, if not by all women, that their presence is absolutely necessary to the existence of this state. In reference to one or two of these signs, this is far from the fact; for they are not unfrequently absent, although pregnancy exist, and the remainder may be present, although pregnancy be absent. Many a female, I am confident, has, from this very circumstance, experienced much difficulty in attaining certainty as to her state, and suffered months of anxiety and doubt. This has arisen from a want of those clear notions, and that precise information, which a question so important demands.

The object of this chapter is to remove this difficulty, by presenting a short account of those symptoms of conception which the female may herself observe, and to point out to what extent they may be relied on. It will be necessary to notice only *four* of the signs or symptoms of pregnancy, and they may be considered in the order in which they usually arise; that is, ceasing to be unwell; morning sickness; shooting pains through, enlargement of, and other changes of the breast; and, lastly, quickening.

Ceasing to be unwell.

The first symptom of pregnancy is the omission of that monthly return, which, in female phraseology, would be described as "ceasing to be unwell;" and it may be adopted as a general rule, that, in a healthy woman, whose menstruation has been established, and continued regular, and who is not nursing, "Conception is followed by a suppression of the menstrual discharge at the next return of its period." Thus, a female may have been pregnant a week or two already; but she is not aware of it till that period of the month arrives when she is accustomed to menstruate, and then, when she expects to be unwell, she finds that she is not so.

Now this symptom, as a general rule, admits of four exceptions:—

First. A young female shall never have menstruated, and yet conceive.

Secondly. A mother shall conceive while she is nursing, and not menstruating.

Thirdly. A female shall conceive, and yet be unwell during the first three, four, or more months of pregnancy.

Fourthly, and lastly. Occasional conception takes place late in life, after menstruation has apparently ceased for ever.

First Exception.—Many cases are on record proving this point. I have met with only two cases; one quite a girl, not having arrived at her seventeenth year, and yet was in her sixth month of pregnancy when she applied for a letter for the Finsbury Midwifery Institution; the other was in her nineteenth year. Menstruation was, subsequent to confinement, established in the first; with the result of the latter, I am not acquainted.*

* A remarkable case is mentioned by Morgagni:—"I was acquainted," he says, "with a maiden of a noble family, who married before menstruation took place, though the menses had been expected for some years; nevertheless she became exceedingly fruitful. We were the less surprised at this circumstance because the same thing had happened to her mother.

Frank attended a patient who gave birth to three children without ever having been unwell. Capuron, also

Although pregnancy under such circumstances is not of frequent occurrence, still it does now and then take place. A knowledge of the fact may therefore prove useful.

Second Exception.—It is scarcely necessary to advert to the well-known fact that a woman may conceive while she is nursing, without any previous return of the monthly discharge, except to expose the popular error, " that a female will not become pregnant during lactation." This is very far from being the case. Poor women are much in the habit of nursing their infants eighteen months, two years, and even two years and a half, in or-

refers to several cases of this description, and Fodere assures us of the fact. A case of the kind occurred too in the practice of Mr. Montgomery. Low likewise mentions a similar instance. Sir E. Moore relates the case of a young woman who married before she was seventeen, and never having menstruated, became pregnant, and four months after delivery was pregnant a second time; the same thing occurred again, and after the third pregnancy she menstruated for the first time, continued to do so for several periods, and became pregnant again.

It should be remembered, however, that some women are very irregular in the return of their menstrual periods—having them prolonged much beyond the usual interval. Mr. Montgomery once attended an unmarried woman of forty, who assured him that returns of the menses had frequently been delayed more than six months without causing ill health. Instances of menstrual suppression for shorter periods are frequent. Zacchias mentions that he attended a patient who used to menstruate regularly, but who never conceived until the discharge had been suppressed for three or four months previously. Mauriceau relates a somewhat similar case, and remarks that cases of this character give rise to the supposition of protracted pregnancy.

der to protect themselves, as they imagine, from becoming pregnant; and many a poor creature have I seen with exhausted frame and disordered general health, arising from protracted nursing, pursued alone from this mistaken notion.

I have large opportunities of investigating this, as well as the several points touched upon in this chapter. On an average, between forty and fifty poor women call upon me every month, with midwifery letters for attendance in their confinement: and the result of my inquiries upon the present question has led me to believe, that more than one third of these women have conceived at least once while nursing, and very many of them oftener.*

Mrs. M——, ætat. 30, married six years. Became pregnant three months after her marriage. Having suckled this child for more than two years, became pregnant a second time. This last died in three weeks, and immediately after she proved pregnant for a third time. The third child she brought this morning (being out of health), and assured me that she had not seen anything since she first conceived, that is, three months after her marriage, and six years from the present time.

Mrs. W——, ætat. 25, married five years. Has not been unwell since she first fell in the

* The following cases, as well as others, are extracted from my Note Book.

family way; is now pregnant with a third child, having hitherto fallen pregnant while nursing.

Many other cases illustrative of this fact I might assert, but these suffice to prove the xception.*

Third Exception.—That a female should become pregnant, and yet be unwell during the first three, four, or more months of pregnancy, may appear an extraordinary statement; but it is a fact, that the menstrual discharge sometimes continues in its usual regularity for two, three, or more months after conception, and without any dangerous consequences.

It has been asserted, as an objection, that this discharge is not truly menstruation; but the discussion of that question does not concern us here. We have only to consider, whether there does not frequently, during pregnancy, take place a discharge, so closely resembling menstruation in its periods, quantity, duration, and appearance, that neither the female herself nor her medical adviser shall be able to detect any difference between them; and of this I have no doubt.

It may occur *once* only after conception, either in diminished quantity or more profuse

* Mr. Robertson of Manchester inquired minutely into the result of one hundred and sixty cases, in which he found that eighty-one women had become pregnant once or oftener during suckling.

than usual. It may thus give rise to miscalculation as to the expected time of confinement.

It may continue in its usual regularity for *two* or *three months.* The following instance of a patient I attended illustrates the fact of its going on to the period of quickening:—

Mrs. R——, ætat. 27, married eight years. Was first unwell when eighteen years of age, and continued to be so regularly until she became pregnant, two years from the time of her marriage. She suckled her first child for eleven months; soon after she became unwell, and continued so until she quickened with her second child; a circumstance which she had not the slightest suspicion of, for there was no perceptible difference either in the quantity or appearance of the monthly discharge. During the remaining months of gestation she did not see anything; she afterwards suckled her little one for ten months; and then was obliged to wean the child, having an attack of the cholera. She continued from this time regular for two years; but meeting with a fall, much to her surprise, two or three days after, miscarried of a four months' child. She is now pregnant again, having been regular every month till she quickened, and expects to be confined, Feb. 1836

In this case then, the female was unwell in two pregnancies till the period of quickening; and in the other for four months, when miscarriage took place from accident.

And lastly, it may occur through the *whole* period of pregnancy.

Mrs. F—— is now pregnant for the third time. In her first pregnancy the monthly returns appeared for three periods, regular as to time, and in quantity and appearance as heretofore. During the second child-bearing, at every month till confinement. During the third—her present pregnancy—for three months only. This patient is always unwell while nursing.

Mrs. J——, now in her eighth pregnancy. Was unwell every month throughout the first six pregnancies; but the quantity always slightly diminished. In the seventh, the same circumstances occurred; but premature labour was this time induced, between the sixth and seventh months, by a fall. During the present pregnancy she has not seen anything. Is always unwell while suckling.

Mrs. P—— is in her fourth pregnancy. In the first three was unwell, at her regular periods, to the time of confinement. The discharge the same in quantity, but rather lighter appearance. Has been unwell in her pregnancy every month up to the present time.*

* Dr. Heberden was acquainted with a lady who never ceased to have regular returns of the menses during four pregnancies, quite to the time of her delivery.—*Heberden Commentaries.*

This opinion is confirmed by Gardien, Dewees, Hamilton, Desormeaux, Puzos, Francis, &c.

The following case proves how important it is that this fact should be generally known; for up to a very late period, some medical men have even denied the possibility of this occurrence.

The case I refer to was that of a young lady, privately married, the gradual enlargement of whose abdomen was decided by her medical attendant to arise from dropsy; for, although she had most of the symptoms of pregnancy, and the medical man was aware she had been married eight months, still, as *she continued to menstruate*, he declared it impossible that she could be pregnant. Tapping was proposed; and, except that her general health suffered much at this time, the operation would have been performed. The delay saved the patient such unfortunate and mistaken treatment—it might have proved fatal in its results—and she shortly gave birth to a living and healthy male child.

Fourth exception.—That women late in life have conceived after menstruation had apparently ceased for ever, the following cases prove:—

In September, 1834, I was called to the assistance of a female in labour in her forty-ninth year. She had not been pregnant for twelve years, and supposed she had ceased to menstruate two years previous to that time. She did well, and never afterward saw anything.

Mrs. B——, ætat. 39. Has been married

eighteen years, commenced to be unwell very early in life. Has had three children; the last pregnancy seven years since. Is now again pregnant, her menses having left her sixteen weeks prior to conception; before which, she had been very irregular, and supposed she had ceased to be unwell for ever.

Other cases of a similar nature are on record. There can be no doubt they are authentic; but at the same time it must be acknowledged that a female is not unlikely to be deceived, by the irregularity which attends the returns of this discharge, late in life. It so happens, too, that just before the change of life takes place, there appears in the constitution of some females a great disposition to pregnancy; so that many who have ceased to bear children for years, or have been hitherto barren through the whole of their married existence, at this time, to the surprise of their friends and themselves, become pregnant.*

* "A woman came to me one morning," says Dr. Gooch, "with a note from a medical man, containing the following statement: The patient's age was forty-two; she had been married twenty-two years without ever being pregnant. About seven months ago she had ceased to menstruate; a few months afterwards the abdomen began to enlarge, and was now nearly equal to that of full pregnancy. For several months the practitioner had been using various means for reducing the tumour, but in vain I examined the case, pronounced her pregnant, and seven weeks afterward she brought forth a child at the full time."

Dr Montgomery says: "A lady in her forty-third year, who was married to her present husband twenty

A knowledge of these facts must be useful, as they will tend to allay apprehension at what might be supposed disease, both by the mother and by the hitherto childless woman.

A female must not forget, however, that she may mistake her condition, and that such mistakes are not at all unlikely to arise from the circumstance that the symptoms which naturally accompany the *cessation* of menstruation, much resemble thoseof pregnancy. She passes over the menstrual period;—she is struck with this. Other symptoms are soon manifested; the size increases—the breasts even become swollen and painful—the stomach disordered, and the appetite capricious;—flatulence collects in the intestines; and while on this account the size still increases, the air moving about the bowels gives an in-

years ago, remained without any promise of offspring until within the last few months; but having missed her menstruation in September last, and finding her size increasing, I was requested to see her in January, when she exhibited evident symptoms of pregnancy. She was subsequently delivered of a healthy boy, after a natural labor of about four hours."

Mosse, one of the medical officers of the Dublin Lying-in-Hospital in 1775, states, that eighty-four of the women delivered in the Institution under his superintendence were between the ages of forty-one and fifty-four; four of these were in the fifty-first year, and one in her fifty-fourth.

In May, 1816, Mrs. Ashley, wife of John Ashley, grazier, of Frisby, at the age of fifty-four years was delivered of two female children.

The succession to an estate was disputed in France because the mother was fifty-eight years old when the child was born. The decision was in favour of the fact ward sensation which is mistaken by the female for the plunging of the child. Time alone, or the investigation of the medical attendant, detects the mistake ; and the symptoms are then to be easily removed by the exhibition of carminative and purgative medicines, the use of active exercise, and bandaging the distended abdomen.

It must be remembered, also, that *suppression* of the monthly return may arise from a variety of causes, altogether independent of conception. Every female is aware, that exposure to cold, just before the expected period, is a frequent cause. Different forms of disease, hardship, or mental emotions, may produce the same result. It does not follow, therefore, because a woman ceases to menstruate, she *must* be pregnant ; which naturally presents this inquiry : what dependence, then, is to be placed upon the omission of menstruation as a symptom or sign of pregnancy ?

When a female ceases to be unwell, and experiences other symptoms of pregnancy, she must consider her situation as yet uncertain, because these signs are common to disease as well as pregnancy. But if toward the third month, while the suppression continues, she recovers her health, and if her appetite and colour return, she needs no better proof of pregnancy ; for under other circumstances her health would remain impaired and even become worse.*

Morning Sickness.

Soon after conception, the stomach often becomes affected with what is called "morning sickness." On first awaking, the female feels as well as usual, but on rising from her bed qualmishness begins, and perhaps while in the act of dressing, retching takes place.

This symptom may occur almost immediately after conception; but it most frequently commences for the first time between two or three weeks after. Now and then it is experienced only the last six weeks or two months of pregnancy, when it is attended, generally, with much distress and discomfort. And lastly, it is not unfrequently absent alto gether.

It continues, more or less, during the first half of pregnancy, and subsides about the time when the movements of the child begin to be felt.

Irritability of the stomach, however, may arise from a variety of causes totally independent of pregnancy, and connected with disease or disordered function. Of what

* It may, however, be considered almost a settled fact, that when a female has menstruated regularly up to the time of cohabitation, and immediately after ceases to menstruate at the time of their usual return, especially if attended with morning sickness—that pregnancy has taken place.

avail, then, it will be asked, is this symptom as a sign of pregnancy? It is so far available:—

The nausea and vomiting of pregnancy are not accompanied by any other symptom of ill health; but, on the contrary, the patien feels as well as ever in other respects, and perchance takes her meals with as much relish as formerly; but while doing so, or immediately after, she feels suddenly sick, and has hardly time to retire, when she rejects the whole contents of her stomach, and very shortly after is quite well again. Not so with sickness arising from disease, or disordered condition of the stomach.

Shooting pains through—enlargement of—and other changes of the breast.

When two months of pregnancy have been completed, an uneasy sensation of throbbing and stretching fulness is experienced, accompanied with tingling about the middle of the breasts, centring in the nipple. A sensible alteration in their appearance soon follows: they grow larger and more firm. The nipple becomes more prominent, and the circle around its base altered in color and structure, constituting what is called "the areola." And, as pregnancy advances, milk is secreted.

The period of gestation at which these changes may occur, as well as the degree in which they become manifested, varies very much. Sometimes, with the exception of the secretion of the milk, they are recognised very soon after conception;—in other instances, particularly in females of a weakly and delicate constitution, they are hardly perceptible until pregnancy is far advanced, or even drawing towards its termination.

Enlargement of the Breast.—The changes in the *form* and *size* of the breast may be the result of causes unconnected with pregnancy. They may enlarge in consequence of marriage, from the individual becoming stout and fat, or from accidental suppression of the monthly return. There are, however, these differences: enlargement from pregnancy may in general be distinguished from that produced merely from fat, by the greater firmness of the breast, and its knotty uneven feeling—it is heavier; and the tension and enlargement from suppressed menstruation, by its subsiding in two or three days, whereas that caused by pregnancy continues to increase. Nevertheless, the dependence which may be placed upon the enlargement of the breast only, as an evidence of pregnancy, is not very great, and considered alone, but a doubtful sign.

The Nipple.—Not so the changes which take place in the nipple, and around its base. These alterations, if present, are of the utmost value, as an evidence of pregnancy. The changes referred to are these:—

About the sixth or seventh week after conception has taken place, if the nipple be examined, it will be found becoming turgid and prominent, and a circle forming around its base, of a colour deeper in its shade than rose or flesh-colour, slightly tinged with a yellowish or brownish hue, and here and there upon its surface will be seen little prominent points, from about ten to twenty in number. In the progress of the next six or seven weeks, these changes are fully developed; the nipple becoming more prominent and turgid than ever: the circle around it of larger dimensions, of an extent of about an inch or an inch and a half; the skin being soft, bedewed with a slight degree of moisture, frequently staining the linen in contact with it; the little prominences of larger size, from the sixteenth to the twelfth of an inch perhaps; and the colour of the whole very much deepened, but always modified by the complexion of the individual, being darker in persons with dark hair, dark eyes, and sallow skins, than in those of fair hair, light-coloured eyes, and delicate complexions.

Such are the essential characteristics of the true areola, the result of pregnancy, and, I believe, of that condition only.

This, then, is a most valuable sign; but, unfortunately, it is frequently absent; and how often it is present, although I have examined many hundred cases for it, I cannot determine, as unfortunately no note was made upon this point. It should also be observed, that both in dark and fair women, the change of colour, without the other appearances, may be present, and yet pregnancy exist; and I have also seen frequently the dark circle alone, where pregnancy did not exist; but I never saw an instance where these prominences were truly developed, without the presence of pregnancy.

This fact has been more particularly noticed of late years by an eminent physician-accoucheur, and the attention of the author has, in consequence, been much directed to it; and, as a striking illustration of its truth, he may mention, that, called upon very recently to visit one of the Institution patients, the third day after her delivery, and having occasion to examine the breast, I pointed out to the gentleman in attendance the presence of these little prominences around the base of the nipple; upon which the patient, to my great surprise, immediately observed, "Ah, sir, I always know when I am pregnant by them, for they appear about ten days or a fortnight after its occurrence, and subsequent to delivery diminish gradually, as my milk leaves me."

It has occurred to me during the past year to be consulted in five cases of doubtful pregnancy. In *two* of them, circumstances forbade the probability of its occurrence; but in both the true areola was distinctly and fully developed. It decided my opinion; and the result proved its correctness: both became mothers. *Two others* had made themselves patients of the Lying-in-Institution, having obtained letters for attendance from governors of the charity, and upon which was marked, by their own calculation, the month of their expected confinement. But I was led to believe, from observing two or three symptoms, that pregnancy did not exist.

Their cases were examined, and at last the breast; in both the true areola was wanting: the review of symptoms decided all doubts. Had, however, the true areola been present in either, it would at once have reversed, instead of confirming my first suspicions.

The *fifth* was pregnant, but the true areola was wanting; and I was obliged to refer to those signs which can alone be recognised by a medical man.

The absence, then, of this sign, except in combination with other circumstances, proves nothing, but, if present, I believe it conclusive.

The Presence of Milk.—With regard to the presence of milk in the breasts, as this is a symptom which may arise, and does very generally, in the latter months of gestation alone, when the existence of pregnancy has been long determined, it is only mentioned here to refute the popular error, that "the presence of milk in the breasts is an infallible proof of pregnancy." It is no such thing; and many well-recorded instances could be brought forward to prove the possibility of its formation under circumstances totally independent of pregnancy.

Belloc speaks of a servant girl, who being obliged to have sleeping with her an infant who was being weaned, and which by its crying disturbed her rest, bethought her of giving it her breast to appease its clamour; and the result was, that in a short time she had milk enough to satisfy the child.*

The following case is related by Mr. George Semple: Mrs. B——, wife of John Breward, Simpson Green, near Idle, aged forty-nine, the mother of nine children, the youngest of whom is twelve years old, lost a daughter-in-law about a year ago, who died in about a fortnight after giving birth to her first child. On her death, Mrs. B. took charge of the infant, a little puny sickly baby. The child was so fretful and uneasy, that Mrs. B. after many sleepless nights, was induced to permit the child to take her nipple into its mouth. In the course of from thirty to thirty-six hours she felt very unwell; her breasts became extremely painful, considerably increased in size, and soon after, to her utter astonishment, milk was secreted, and poured forth in the same abundance as n former occasions, after the birth of her own children. The child, now a year old, is a fine, thriving, healthy girl, and only a few

* Cours de Méd. Légale, p. 52

days ago I saw her eagerly engaged in obtaining an apparently abundant supply of healthy nourishment, from the same fountain which, nearly twenty years ago, poured forth its resources for the support of her father." *

* North of Eng. Med. and Surg. Journ., vol. i., p. 230.

That the presence of milk in the female breast shall take place independent of pregnancy, from the above and other recorded facts, there can be no doubt; but the following beautiful exemplification of its formation in that of the *male*, places the question in a still stronger light. This interesting fact is cited from Captain Franklin's narrative of his journey to the shores of the Polar Sea.

"A young Chipewyan had separated from the rest of his band, for the purpose of entrapping beaver, when his wife, who was his sole companion, and in her first pregnancy, was seized with her pains of labor. She died on the third day, after giving birth to a boy. The husband was inconsolable, and vowed in his anguish, never to take another woman to wife; but his grief was soon in some degree absorbed in anxiety for the fate of his infant son. To preserve its life he descended to the office of a nurse, so degrading in the eyes of a Chipewyan, as partaking of the duties of a woman. He swaddled it in soft moss, fed it with broth made from the flesh of the deer; and to still its cries, applied it to his breast, praying earnestly to the Great Master of Life to assist his endeavors. The force of the powerful passion by which he was actuated produced the same effect in his case as it has done in some others which are recorded: a flow of milk actually took place from his breast. He succeeded in rearing his child, taught him to be a hunter, and when he attained the age of manhood, chose him a wife from the tribe. The old man kept his vow in never taking a wife for himself, but he delighted in tending his son's children; and when his daughter-in-law used to interfere, saying, that it was not the occupation of a man, he was wont to reply, that he had promised the Great Master of Life, if his child was spared, never to be pr[illegible] like other Indians. Our informant, Mr. Wen-

Quickening.

There is only one other symptom which I think it useful to notice, that is quickening; by which is meant, the first sensation experienced by the mother of the *life* of the child within her womb.

The first time this motion of the child occurs, the sensation is like that of the fluttering of a bird within her, and so sudden that she frequently faints, or falls into an hysterical paroxysm. A day or two passes by when it recurs. It afterwards increases both in frequency and degree, until the movements of the child are fully recognised.

It is proper that a female should be informed that the *period* when quickening takes place is very uncertain; for an impression is popularly prevalent that it always occurs *exactly* at the end of four calendar months and a half. This is not the case; it varies in different women, and in the same women during different pregnancies as the following one or two instances will prove:—

Mrs. F——. Quickened with her first child at four months: quickened with the se-

kel (one of the Association) added, that he had often seen this Indian in his old age, and that his left breast, even then, retained the unusual size it had acquired in his occupation of nurse." P. 157.

Man possesses the same organization as woman for secreting and conveying milk, which enables us readily both to understand and believe in the truth of the foregoing singular statement.

cond at fourteen weeks: and is now in her third pregnancy, and reckons from the fourteenth week again.

Mrs. B——. Has had seven children, and with all felt the motion of the child for the first time at the third month.

Mrs. Mc M.——. Has been several times pregnant; seldom feels movements of the child at all until the sixth month, and not strongly till the eighth.

The annexed table of the periods of quickening of seventy cases taken in the order in which they have been entered in the author's note-book, will forcibly stamp the truth of these opinions:

9	Quickened at the 3d month.
11	Quickened at 3½ months.
21	Quickened at the 4th month.
16	Quickened at 4½ months
8	Quickened at the 5th month.
1	Quickened at 5½ months.
4	Quickened at the 6th month.
70	

In a few of these cases, for the sake of convenience I have used round numbers, when two or three days before or after was the exact time, and for the sake of correctness, have omitted several cases, in which there was the slightest doubt in the patient's mind of the exact time.

It appears from this table, that this symp

tom takes place more frequently between the twelfth and sixteenth week, than before or after these periods; and that subsequent to the 4½ and the expiration of the sixth month, it may occur in the proportion of more than one case out of every five.—Before the third month, quickening seldom arises.

This symptom may not be felt by the mother at all, and yet pregnancy exist. This is rare, but the fact is confirmed by many writers; and I have met during the last seven years with two instances, and in both the mothers gave birth to living and healthy children.

Now comes the question, how far this symptom is of value, as a sign of the pregnant state?

If it has been experienced in former pregnancies, it is invaluable, for I believe it is not to be mistaken. If it is a first pregnancy and doubtful, it removes all obscurity, provided the sensation grows stronger and stronger, until the movements of the child are distinctly felt.

Four only of the symptoms of pregnancy have been noticed, because the remainder are not recognisable, except by the accoucheur, although to him of the greatest value when pregnancy is complicated and doubtful from the presence of disease.

The nature of these symptoms has been described as plainly, and yet as briefly, as possible, because of the importance of their being clearly understood by married women.

I have also endeavored to point out their real value as evidence of pregnancy—how they are sometimes absent in patients who are pregnant, and some of them present in those who are not so—because of the doubt and obscurity which arise from these variations.

And lastly, in bringing these observations to a conclusion, I venture to say, that if the married female will only take the trouble to make herself familiar with this little detail, she will not regret the time as lost or mis-spent, because it will generally guide her aright, and I trust save her many moments of anixety and discomfort.

ON THE

DISEASES OF PREGNANCY,

AND HINTS FOR THEIR

PREVENTION AND RELIEF.

In describing the diseases which are incident to the whole period of pregnancy, my design is to take a general popular survey of the subject. I wish simply to communicate that kind of information, which every married and well-educutad woman should certainly possess, and can usefully employ. To advance further than this, to those points upon which the assistance of the medical adviser ought to be sought, would be on every account improper, and productive rather of evil than of good.

There is no organ in the body, with the exception of the stomach, that exercises a more extensive control over the female system than the womb. Hence, when in the condition of pregnancy, it affects, directly or indirectly, various parts of that system. The effects of pregnancy, however, vary much according to the constitution of the female.

Sometimes a very salutary change is produced, so that the individual enjoys better health during gestation than before. The delicate and frequent-ailing girl, for instance, —the propriety of whose marrying was a matter of doubt among her friends—becoming pregnant, instead of realizing the apprehensions and fears of those most dear to her will sometimes acquire new life and vigor from the altered circumstances of her condition. On the other hand, speaking generally it is sometimes the case that harassing and painful symptoms will arise. These are designated the "diseases of pregnancy."

Morning Sickness.

Nausea or vomiting, is one of the most common and distressing affections of pregnancy. It is chiefly troublesome in the earlier months of gestation, continuing until the period of quickening, when it decreases or ceases spontaneously;—or it does not occur until the latter months of pregnancy, when it subsides only upon delivery. I shall consider these states separately; and—

First, of sickness during the *earlier* months.

This arises solely from sympathy with the newly commenced action, and irritable condition of the womb. This is evident from the fact, that, as the novelty of the pregnant state ceases, and the stomach becomes accustomed to it, the sickness subsides gradually, and is rarely troublesome afterwards.

It occasionally commences immediately after conception; and it is a remarkable fact, that a pregnant woman scarcely ever feels sick, until she first gets upon her feet in the morning. Hence it is called the "morning sickness." She awakes refreshed and well arises from her bed, and while dressing begins to feel qualmish. At the breakfast table she has no appetite, or if she takes anything, is shortly obliged to leave for her dressing-room, where she returns what she has taken; or, if she has been unable to take anything, ejects a fluid, limpid, thin and watery; and if the vomiting increases in severity, bile is thrown up at the same time. After the lapse of three or four hours, she feels quite well again, and by dinner time sits down with an appetite to her meal.

If there is merely nausea or vomiting *without the presence of bile*, it is evident that it arises solely from irritability of the stomach, and is not connected with a disordered condition of the digestive organs, which latter circumstance is not unfrequently the case. The best means that can be employed to relieve this irritable state will be found in a draught taken twice a day for several days, composed of fifteen grains of magnesia, one drachm of tincture of columba, and an ounce and a half of distilled peppermint-water.*

Medicine sometimes is hardly called for · and I have known a tumbler of warm chamomile tea, or even warm water only, taken immediately after nausea was felt, by inducing immediate vomiting, tranquillize the disturbed stomach, and thus abridge the morning attack. It is sometimes attended with advantage to take the chamomile tea before the female rises from her bed. I advised this with the most marked success very lately in the case of a lady who was very much reduced by the morning sickness. It had continued for several weeks, and with so much violence and straining, as to cause blood to be ejected with the fluid. In less than one week, when all other means had previously failed, the above suggestion was successful.

It frequently happens that the acidity is very great, in which case fifteen or twenty grains of magnesia should be taken in a wine-glass of milk*—or, if it is preferred, a

* I have found a Burgundy pitch plaster, the surface of which has been well sprinkled with powdered opium, an admirable application to the pit of the stomach. In many cases the nausea has been soon relieved, and the irritability of the stomach subdued.

* A teaspoonful of pulverized prepared charcoal in a

small tumbler of soda water; but the latter must not be persevered in for any great length of time, as it will then become injurious. The presence of acidity, however, is sometimes so difficult to overcome by alkalies, that these medicines must be given up, and acid remedies employed. Lemonade may first be taken, but lemon-juice and water is still better.

The state of the bowels must not be forgotten, and if any of the latter remedies are resorted to, the most marked benefit will be derived from a gentle dose of Epsom or Cheltenham salts every second morning, if so often necessary.†

The diet in such a case must also be carefully attended to; but as this point will be referred to more particularly presently, it is only necessary now to say that the quantity of food taken must bear some proportion to the slightly diminished powers of the digestive functions, and that it will be well, when the sickness is very obstinate and distressing, to take no food at all for several hours after rising. If, after a few hours, the mouth is

tablespoonful of lime water, is oftentimes very useful in these cases.

† Seidlitz powders with a little syrup of ginger are frequently efficient, particularly if followed by a large draught of pure water. Many who have taken the Seidlitz powders with little or no effect, would be surpr se at their efficacy, if one or two tumblers of water be taken immediately afterwards.

much parched, it may be moistened with a little broth, or weak beef-tea; but let nothing more be taken for five or six hours, and it is most probable that the sickness which has resisted all other means, will thus be relieved.

If this irritable state of the stomach is connected with a *disordered condition* of the *digestive organs*, the sickness will be accompanied with the presence of bile in the matter vomited, a furred tongue, confined or irregular action of the bowels, and occasionally with what is termed "a sick headache." These symptoms are to be relieved by medicines which thoroughly clear out the bowels, allay the irritability of the stomach, and afterwards by those which restore tone to both. But it is to be observed that the following directions are only intended to apply to those simple cases, in which, whether necessary or not, no one ever thinks of consulting their medical adviser, and for which it is certainly desirable that they should have some judicious directions, rather than be left entirely without them. If these symptoms become at all aggravated, it is requisite that they should make immediate application for professional advice.

The bowels will need in the first instance a draught composed of infusion of senna and Epsom salts—the common "black draught,"—with half a drachm of the tincture of hen bane in addition. This, with five grains of blue pill, most probably effects the object desired; the bowels will be well purged, and the tongue become clean.

The next thing is to allay the irritability of the stomach, which is to be accomplished by the means already pointed out—the effervescing draught of soda, magnesia, chamomile tea, &c.; but in connexion with this, two or three grains of the purified extract of aloes, with an equal quantity of the extract of henbane, must be taken two or three times a week, at bedtime. This will keep the tongue still clean, and the bowels in order.

After a little time, the sickness having subsided, tonic medicines may be used: and a fourth part of the following mixture, taken three times a day, will, under the present circumstances, be the best means of restoring the tone of the stomach and bowels: sulphate of quinine, six grains; diluted sulphuric acid, half a drachm; infusion of columba, five ounces and a half; simple syrup, half an ounce.

Having pointed out the means for mitigating sickness in the early months, there only remains one additional suggestion to make, and it is, that all the remedies for relief detailed may, in some cases, fail. The sickness continues most obstinate; every time the female takes food, or even sometimes when abstaining from it, she vomits; and at last, from this excessive irritability and long continued violent action of the stomach, symptoms threatening miscarriage will manifest themselves.* There is generally in such a case, pain and a sensation of tension about the pit of the stomach, increased after every attack of sickness. If symptoms of miscarriage are not present, the application of nine or twelve leeches to the stomach, and pieces of soft linen rag well soaked with laudanum, constantly applied and renewed, will give the most decided relief. If, however, there is pain in the loins and hips, increasing in frequency and power, becoming at last slightly bearing down, I strongly advise the patient to consult her medical adviser, as the loss of a little blood from the arm, perfect rest in the recumbent position, and other directions which he alone can give, will, in such a case, be absolutely necessary, and I may add, if perseveringly acted up to by the patient herself, be certainly followed by success.

Secondly, of sickness coming on at the *conclusion* of pregnancy.

This arises from the distended state of the womb affecting mechanically, by its pressure, the coats of the stomach, and certain parts of its neighborhood.

This form of vomiting but rarely occurs

* In these cases, the oil of kreosote will be found a most valuable remedy. It is given in doses of from half a drop to one drop. This medicine, however, ought not to be used without the sanction of a medical man.

for do not let me be supposed to refer to the sickness which sometimes immediately precedes, and generally accompanies, the early part of labour. I am speaking of that irritability of the stomach which may arise about the sixth, seventh, or eighth month, and from which the female has been entirely free during the previous months of gestation, and now producing vomiting of an exceedingly troublesome form.

A lady suffering from sickness thus late in pregnancy, ought to seek medical advice at once. From this cause, if severe, premature labour might be brought on, and judicious medical treatment is always decidedly necessary to mitigate this form of sickness. The patient must lose a little blood, she must keep strictly to her sofa, and the bowels ought to be gently acted upon by small doses of Cheltenham or Epsom salts. A grain of the extract of opium may be given to allay the irritability at night, and cloths dipped in laudanum frequently applied to the pit of the stomach.

In all forms of sickness arising from pregnancy as its cause, the diet must be light, mild, and nutritious, taken in moderate quantities of three or four meals a day. It should consist of mild animal food, boiled or roasted. Chicken, white game boiled, mutton or beef roasted, are the viands most nutritious and easily digested. Stale pure bread untoasted, or pilot bread, mealy potatoes, or well-boiled rice, in moderate quantities, may be taken with animal food for dinner. A glass of port wine with warm water at the conclusion of the meal, is the best kind of beverage.

Advantage has often been derived from always taking brown bread, and Jamaica sugar in the morning's coffee. The healthy operation of the bowels has thus been promoted; although a system of regular exercise by walking, apportioned to the strength, and not continued so long as to fatigue, will generally effect this purpose, while at the same time it gives tone to the general health. Fatigue of body is sedulously to be avoided. Slow and moderate walks, exercise in an open carriage (if the patient has sufficient strength), should be taken daily between breakfast and dinner; always avoiding to sit down to the latter meal tired, and, therefore, probably, with a blunted appetite.*

Heartburn.

This is a very distressing symptom, and occurs early after conception; sometimes,

* Besides the morning sickness, the period of pregnancy is often attended with another distressing symptom, described as a sinking at the pit of the stomach: the patient complains, to use a common expression, that she feels *all gone*. This feeling I have often relieved by the free use of soda water. Another remedy which I have often used, and which is by no means disagreeable, is a fresh egg, beaten up with a tumbler of milk, and sweetened

however, not till after the fourth month; and occasionally is absent altogether. It is produced by an acid forming on the stomach, which rises into the throat, and, from the sensation it occasions, is called *heartburn.*

It is a very common complaint of pregancy, and every female knows that she finds relief by taking a little magnesia or chalk, or lime-water and milk, with the occasional use of magnesia; but, although these means generally mitigate this symptom, occasionally it is very severe and almost intractable, and they fail. Under such circumstances, a draught composed of 15 grains of magnesia, 10 drops of the solution of the subcarbonate of ammonia, and 1½ ounce of mint or peppermint-water, taken three times a day, and continued for three or four days, will remove the complaint.

If the bowels are confined, as is frequently the case, mild doses of Epsom or Cheltenham salts will be the best aperients. The use of these must be regulated by circumstances,—taken every second, third, or fourth day that is, resorted to with sufficient frequency and perseverance to guard against costiveness.*

The *diet* must also, in every case, be strictly attended to, and regulated upon the plan already stated.

* The *Red* mixture, prepared by suspending equal parts of pulverized rhubarb and magnesia in mint water. is a favorite prescription with many

Costiveness.

A costive state of bowels is one of the most common and, at the same time, troublesome of the diseases of pregnancy. It arises partly from the increased activity which is going on in the womb, and which induces a slug gish condition of the bowels, and partly from the pressure of the now enlarged and ex panded womb on the bowels themselves.

A confined state of bowels is the frequent source of many serious evils; it therefore behoves the female to be vigilant and guard against it.

First,—Because, as before stated, pregnancy itself predisposes to constipation.

Secondly,—Because it is much more easily prevented than removed, when, after several days' confinement, an accumulation of hardened fœces has collected in the lower bowel.

Thirdly,—Because such an accumulation may give rise to inflammation of the bowel itself, and, in the earlier months of pregnancy, to miscarriage; and,

Lastly,—Because, if a female falls into labor with her intestinal canal so loaded, it will of itself be sufficient to render, what would otherwise have been a quick, easy, and safe labor, a long, painful, and difficult one; and may be the cause also of very serious and alarming symptoms some forty or eight-and-forty hours after her labor is over.

The first and leading symptom of this affection is a costive or more consistent state than usual of the fœcal excretions, with a less frequent call for evacuation than is customary with the individual when in health. If this is not attended to, and several days, perhaps a week, pass by without the bowels being relieved at all, pain in the head, a foul tongue, and an increased degree of fulness and tension of the abdomen, are experienced. These symptoms are followed, in all probability, by thin watery evacuations, attended with pain, weight, and pressure about the lower bowel; they become frequent; and the female at last, finding that the bowels are not only open again, but even loose, takes chalk mixture. She is not aware that this very looseness is nothing more than increased secretion of the lining membrane of the bowel, caused by the pressure of the accumulated mass of hardened fœces, which it passes and leaves unmoved. The chalk mixture relieves the irritation upon which the looseness depends, but the disease is not removed, and, instead of its being a case simply of costiveness, it has now become one of constipation; an accumulation of hardened stool is distending and irritating, by its pressure, the lower bowel and the womb, and the serious consequences before enumerated may follow.

Very often have I been consulted by a female far advanced in pregnancy for what she supposed mere looseness of bowels, which has already been found to originate under circumstances like these. It is of the highest importance that the patient should endeavor to guard against such a result; and without doubt she may avoid it, and regulate her bowels with great comfort to herself, throughout the whole period of pregnancy, if she will only use the means.

In pointing out a plan to accomplish this desirable object, the first prescription I have to offer is by far the most valuable,—"prevention is more easy than cure."* If the bowels are sluggish to-day,—that is to say, if they are not as freely relieved as usual,—and you do not assist them by medicine, depend upon it, to-morrow they will be confined, and there will be no relief at all. If, then, the bowels are *disposed* to be costive, I would recommend one large table-spoonful of castor-oil—if it does not nauseate the stomach,—and advise that the dose be repeated in four hours, if the desired effect has not been produced, or a wine-glass of beaume de vie at night; and early the next morning, before leaving the dressing-room, let the lavement be used, the injection consisting merely of a pint of blood-warm water;—or the following pills will be found useful to be kept in the patient's bed-room:—Two scru-

* In these cases medicine is not always necessary. Much benefit may be derived from the use of a laxative diet. Brown bread, mush, or hasty-pudding made from rye or Indian meal, and eaten with molasses, the free use of the dried laxative fruits, as figs, dates, stewed prunes, and our native fruits when ripe, will often enable the patient to dispense with medicine

ple of the compound extract of colocynth and one of the extract of henbane divided into twelve pills. Two or three of these may be taken at bedtime, when the bowels have not been, during the day, satisfactorily relieved. These are always ready in the bedroom, and, as they generally answer the object efficiently, and with comfort to the patient, are the most convenient form of aperient.

It will now and then happen, however, that the female has let the day slip. When this is the case, in combination with medicine, the use of the lavement is desirable. Medicine alone will not answer the purpose, unless it be taken in doses so strong as will not only move the bowels but irritate them too. With the exhibition of the warm water, mild aperients never fail. Females, generally, are averse to the use of the lavement, and it is a prejudice which is most deeply to be regretted. I have known purgative medicines so often resorted to, and, in time, so increased in power and quantity, because they began to lose their effect, that, by their continual irritation disease of the lower bowel has been produced, and death has, at last, been the consequence. If, then, the bowels have been one or two days confined, the lavement in the morning will render much less medicine necessary, and frequently have an effect when medicine alone would not. Many ladies use the warm water every second or third morning, during the latter weeks of pregnancy; and by this means they regulate their bowels—which would otherwise be confined—with great comfort to themselves, and need no medicine at all.

I will only add one word, in conclusion, upon this subject. Let it be remembered, that if the bowels have been confined several days, and diarrhœa comes on, that this is not a natural relief, but the effect of irritation, caused by the presence of a loaded state of the lower bowel, which must be quickly removed by the medical attendant, or it may give rise to some one of those serious evils already enumerated.

Diarrhœa.

An affection very opposite to that which has just been discussed, may occur during pregnancy. We have seen how diarrhœa may arise as a symptom of costiveness. It will manifest itself, however, independently of such a cause. The intestines may participate in the irregularity of the womb, and, their vermicular action becoming morbidly increased, diarrhœa is the consequence. It is a disease which varies very much in differen individuals, and may clearly be divided intc two kinds.

One, in which the motions are more loose and frequent than in health, but not otherwise much altered in their appearance. The tongue is clean, or only slightly white, and the appetite is pretty good. No medicine is required here; a careful diet will correct the evil.

In the other case, the stools are liquid dark-coloured, and very offensive, accompanied with a coated tongue, bad taste, offensive breath, loss of appetite, and more or less disorder of the digestive organs. In these latter circumstances, your medical adviser should be consulted; in case you do not see him, I have found at first the following draught, given every three or four hours, very useful;—rhubarb, eight grains; ipecacuanha, one grain; dill water, one ounce.

As the tongue cleans, the stool becomes more natural, a wine-glass, three times a day, of some bitter infusion, such as cascarilla, orange peel, or gentian, may be taken with advantage. If the diarrhœa continues for any length of time, it is always wise to have the surface of the body kept warm with flannel; and this is best accomplished by a flannel roller bound gently round the abdomen.

But in either form of this disease, whatever remedies are proposed, there is one mode of treatment applicable to both, and which is the most important of all; a proper system of *diet*. The food must be sparing in quantity, of the mildest quality, and such as to leave, after the process of digestion, as little excrementitious matter as possible.

In a recent attack, the *first* day, the patient should only take mild drinks, containing a small quantity of unirritating nutriment; such as barley-water, or arrowroot made with water. Irish moss will be found palable. During the *next* day or *two* the same iet must be continued, but may be given in larger qnantity, and of greater strength. Tapioca, sago, and rice-gruel might be added to the list. When the irritation is somewhat allayed, on the *third* or *fourth* day, perhaps, broth may be taken; but no solid food of any kind, least of all solid animal food, until the disease is removed or greatly allayed. As soon as this is the case, a small quantity of the lightest animal food may be taken; such as the animal jellies, made from calves' head or feet, chicken with well-boiled rice, white game boiled, roast mutton and beef may follow; but lamb and veal for the future should be avoided.

It may be observed, that in some cases, where the diarrhœa has been of long standing, a *drier* diet is best, the liquid food appearing to keep up the disease. Rice well boiled, and merely moistened with a little broth, is the best and one of the most desirable articles of diet in such cases.

Piles.

Pregnant women are very subject to piles. Both with costiveness and diarrhœa they are a frequent attendant, but particularly with the former. They will usually disappear, if they are slight, as soon as the bowels are restored to a healthy action ; but they may not, and then will give rise to great suffering.

The pregnant woman recognises piles under two forms : 1, where they exist as little tumours within or without the bowel, becoming, very soon after their exclusion, more solid and firm, unless they early break and bleed ; and 2, where they present, without the bowel, a tumour, large in circumference, separable in lobes, altogether like a piece of sponge coloured, and bleeding occasionally from the surface.

Of all the *causes* which operate in the production of piles, habitual constipation is the most frequent. The excrementitious matter is delayed in the bowel, becomes hard and knotty, and a source of great irritation: this irritation induces a determination of blood to the part, and the gradual dilatation of its vessels takes place as a consequence, which eventually forms the tumours known under the appellation of *piles*. Now, as in pregnancy there is a greater disposition to costiveness than at any other time, and as piles are a consequence of this disordered function, so this disease is much more prevalent during the pregnant state than at any other period ; another argument, and a very powerful one, why costiveness should be dili gently guarded against.

The *symptoms* of this complaint are well known. There will be weight, heat, and a sense of fulness about the lower bowel, a frequent desire both to relieve the bowels and bladder; all of which symptoms are removed for a time if a discharge of blood takes place.

If the piles be without the bowel, they are constantly irritated by the friction of the parts in the ordinary motion and erect position of the body, and that to a painful degree during the period of the evacuation of the bowels. If exercise be taken in a carriage, the pain is much aggravated; and if the irritation produce inflammation, the piles will become swollen, red or purple, and excessively painful.

The *treatment* of this disease, when it occurs during pregnancy, is two-fold—general and local. We must remove the *cause* by such means as excite a brisker action of the bowels; and our choice of aperients must be directed to those which act efficiently but mildly, and without irritating the lower bowel itself.* Next to small and repeated doses of castor oil—say a table-spoonful,—

* Mild lavements or enemata are here highly serviceable. Where the excrementitious matter is hardened or compacted, the distension of the bowels by from a quart to three pints of starch water, followed by weak soap suds, is a very efficient remedy

he most desirable form of aperient that can be employed is the confection of senna, that is, lenitive electuary, combined with sulphur and magnesia. Of the following form, a dessert-spoonful or more should be taken, at first, twice daily :—Confection of senna, two ounces ; flowers of sulphur, one ounce ; carbonate of magnesia, two drachms and a half. In conjunction with this medicine, much benefit may be derived by the injection of half a pint of warm or cold water—whichever soothes most—as a lavement ; but it must be administered very cautiously, to avoid irritating the parts with the pipe of the instrument.

It is important that medicine, in frequent use, should be so taken as to act upon the bowels in the evening only ; for if the bowels are acted upon in the morning, the patient being obliged to move about all day, will suffer considerable distress and local irritation ; whereas, if the bowels are not evacuated till the evening, the horizontal position, and the perfect rest of a long night, will obviate all inconvenience.

Great assistance may be afforded in the cure, and also in alleviating pain, by external applications to the tumours themselves. If, however, the piles are swollen and inflamed, and the pain experienced great, half a dozen leeches, or from half a dozen to a dozen, should be first applied in their immediate neighbourhood, the parts fomented, and then warm bread and water poultices renewed every three hours.

These remedies will afford very considerable relief; and, when the inflamed state is subdued, an ointment must be applied to the tumours and around them night and morning, composed of two drachms of powdered galls, half a drachm of camphor, and two ounces of lard; or composed of one drachm of powdered black hellebore root, rubbed down in one ounce of lard. The latter preparation will, for some time after its application, give much pain, but proportionate relief will follow.

The *diet* must be sparing in quantity, mild in quality, and such as to leave after its digestion, as little to pass through the bowels as possible.

I would beg attention to one more observation on this subject. The removal of piles by operation, during the pregnant state, is perhaps never justifiable. Let the patient, therefore, consult her medical attendant in time, and not by a false delicacy expose herself to an evil which it is her duty to endeavour to prevent.

Enlargement of the Veins of the Legs.

This is a frequent, but not very trouble some, accompaniment of the latter months of pregnancy. It arises in some degree from the pressure of the womb upon the large venous trunks, impeding to a certain extent the free flow of blood through them. It is frequently remarked in pregnant women who have passed a certain age; but it is particularly unusual for it to happen, in the case of young women, even during a series of repeated pregnancies.

When first observed, *if the veins have not become knotty*,—that is, having little lumps or swellings in their course up the leg,—the only means which it is necessary to employ, is the application of a muslin or cotton bandage,—six yards in length, and as wide as three fingers—from the sole of the foot up to the knee, and sufficiently firm to give support to the venous trunks. This bandage well and equally applied to the limb, with a little aperient medicine twice a week, and the recumbent position for two or three hours in the middle of the day, will cure this form of the affection.

When after a time the *veins, more and more distended, have become lengthened, tortuous, coiled up or knotty*, the female begins to experience a sense of heaviness, numbness, and sometimes very acute wandering pain, through the whole of the affected limb. In a more advanced stage, in proportion as the knotty tumours increase, the limb becomes generally swollen.

This form of the disease calls for much care and patience on the part of the sufferer. The legs should be strapped, from ankle to knee, with strips of adhesive plaster, and over this a muslin or cotton bandage must be applied with a moderate degree of tightness, and kept wet with goulard water. In conjunction with these local appliances, it is sometimes wise to lose a few ounces of blood from the arm, and always necessary to take every other night a gentle aperient, to live upon a spare diet, and for some days to keep the horizontal posture. An elastic laced stocking made for the purpose may be afterward worn, and will be found at once a sufficient support to the limb, and a source of great comfort to the wearer.

Swelling of the Feet and Legs.

In the course of pregnancy, during the latter months particularly, the feet and legs frequently become much enlarged. It is partly owing to the pressure of the womb, but sometimes apparently independent of it. It is first observed towards night, about the ankles; by degrees the swelling rises higher, and the legs may become of a very large size. The female suffering from this complaint, always goes to bed with legs much swollen, but towards morning her face swells and the enlargement of the legs disappears to a greater or less extent, returning, however, as the day advances.

Sometimes this disease is very trifling in its character, and in ordinary cases, except aperients, no medicine is necessary, and support may be given by a well-applied flannel roller; but when the swelling is extensive and permanent, remaining in the same degree after the patient has been for several hours in bed, and connected with uncomfortable sensations in the head, an accelerated pulse &c., a medical man ought to be consulted, for the consequences might otherwise be dangerous.

Palpitation of the Heart.

If this affection occur for the first time during pregnancy, it is rarely connected with disease of the heart itself; it is therefore without danger, although very distressing. Occasionally there is connected with it throbbing of the vessels in the temples, as also in the abdomen; the latter not unfrequently mistaken by the patient for the beatings of the heart itself.

It will make its attack repeatedly in the course of a day, particularly after a meal; and very frequently at night, on first lying down in bed; and it may be brought on at any time by the slightest agitation of mind.

Treatment for an attack.—When it comes on it is to be relieved by putting the hands and arms up to the elbows in water, as warm as can be borne—friction with the warm hand applied to the feet—absolute rest—and taking the following draught: Compound spirits of ammonia, half a tea-spoonful; Camphor mixture, a wine-glass. It may be repeated again in an hour or so, if necessary. It will be well to keep a bottle of this mixture in the bedroom; a resource will always be then at hand, and the dread which attends anticipation in a great measure removed This is the more necessary, as an attack, if it comes on in the night, is always very distressing. The patient awakes, perhaps, out of a frightful dream, with a sense of fluttering in the region of the heart—calls out for breath —begs to have the curtains of the bed withdrawn, the door of the room opened—and will tell you she feels as if she was dying;—wine, brandy, any stimulant that is at hand is resorted to, for the husband or friend of the patient is naturally much excited, and in his alarm scarcely knows how to act. Now there is no occasion for alarm; the sufferer must be assured of this; her mind must be soothed and quieted; the means just pointed out for the relief of a paroxysm must be used; the palpitation will after a little time cease, and the patient will drop off into a quiet and tranquil sleep.

These attacks may be prevented by taking for ten days or a fortnight a tea-spoonful of the following electuary three times a day:—Carbonate of iron, one ounce and a half syrup of ginger, one ounce and a half. The bowels must be carefully regulated; a table-spoonful of Elixir Prop. is the best aperient, provided there are no piles. Fatigue and al exertion must be avoided, and the mind kept perfectly tranquil.

Fainting Fits.

Fainting may occur at any period of pregnancy; but is most frequent during the first three months, and especially about the time of quickening. It may come on when the person is at perfect rest; but is ordinarily produced by unusual exertion,—exposure to heat,—or any sudden excitement of the mind. The paroxysm or fit is sometimes of short duration; and the female does not lose her recollection; she has a knowledge of what is going on about her, and soon recovers; but in other instances the fainting fit is complete and of long duration, continuing for an hour, or upwards.

The treatment during a fit.—This consists in immediately placing the patient in a recumbent posture—the use of pungent volatiles—sprinkling the face with cold water—free exposure to air, and the cautious administration of cordials. And if the fit continue long, the extremities must be kept warm, and the friction of a warm hand be applied to the feet.

It is scarcely necessary to add, that those who are subject to these attacks ought to avoid fatigue—crowded or hot rooms—fasting too long, quick motion, and agitation of mind. The bowels must be attended to and a wine-glass of the infusion of columbo or cascarilla, taken every morning, will be useful in giving tone to the system.

After a few weeks the disposition to fainting will altogether subside, and although a very alarming state to those who are inexperienced, yet the subject of it should never allow her mind to be depressed, or to anticipate an unfavorable result. Pure air, simple diet, and regular exercise, as we said above, will do much to prevent it.

Toothache.

This may appear a trifling disease, to notice in connexion with the subject before us; but, in the course of pregnancy, females will sometimes suffer severely from erratic pains in the face and teeth. As these pains are generally induced by the increased irritability of the nervous system, the result of the new action which is going on in the womb, and not from the decay of any particular tooth, extraction of any tooth for its cure is out of the question. Indeed, did the suffering arise from a carious tooth, its removal is unadvisable, inasmuch as this operation has been immediately followed by a miscarriage. The fact is, that the patients who have consulted me while suffering from this affection, have had, apparently, in most cases, very sound teeth; and, feeling confident that its cause has been what has been before pointed out, the treatment has been purely constitutional.

The following pill may be taken, night and morning:—Socotrine aloes, one grain and a half; blue pill, two grains; together with one drachm of the rust, or carbonate of iron, mixed with treacle or milk. The latter must be repeated twice a day for four days, and then a third dose may be added in the middle of the day; and the remedy continued, even after all uneasiness in the face has subsided for some time, with great advantage to the general health.

The only local application I would advise, is that of washing out the mouth and teeth, night and morning, with salt and cold, or lukewarm water. This plan of treatment not only relieves the painful affection of the face and teeth, but allays also that local irritability of the nerves, upon which it depended.

If a carious tooth seems alone affected, it has been proposed carefully to apply a drop or two of nitric acid, which is said to be infallible; a drop or two of oil of kreosote or cajeput is frequently useful.

Salivation.

A pregnant female must not be surprised, f, some little time after conception, or during any of the months of gestation, the ordinary quantity of saliva, which lubricates and keeps the mouth constantly moist, should increase to such an extent as to be exceedingly troublesome; and, indeed, sometimes become so excessive, as seriously to affect her health. It is a symptom of pregnancy. but a very unusual one; although the quantity of saliva discharged has now and then exceeded three, and even four pints daily.

It differs essentially from the salivation produced by the exhibition of mercury, inasmuch as in this case, there is no tenderness of the gums, or disagreeable fœtor in the breath. The fluid itself is either perfectly colorless and transparent, or more tenacious and frothy. It has an unpleasant taste, and, when tenacious, induces vomiting. It is generally accompanied with acidity; and the plan of *treatment* most advisable, when the disease is moderate in its character, is the frequent use of from twenty to thirty grains of magnesia, say every morning, rinsing the mouth out very often with lime-water, and to resist the desire to discharge the saliva from the mouth as much as possible, for, if it is not very great in quantity, it may be swallowed to advantage. Should this symptom, however, be very excessive, the health will suffer considerably in consequence, and the assistance of the medical man is imperatively called for.

A Painful and Distended Condition of the Breasts.

Pain and tension of the breasts frequently

attend, as also they are natural consequences of, conception.

In a first pregnancy, a large and rapid development of this organ may take place, the breast becoming two or three times as large as before marriage; but if tight lacing be only avoided, and the breasts be permitted to expand, no material inconvenience will arise from this circumstance.

As, however, these symptoms are sometimes attended with considerable distress, I would advise, under such circumstances, the application of half a dozen leeches, or more, tepid fomentations, and a gentle aperient—two drachms of Epsom salts in a little peppermint water—night and morning. These means, by relieving the over distension and fulness of the vessels of the part, remove the cause and complaint at once.

If these symptoms occur to a female who may have been several times pregnant, and formerly has had an abscess in one or other breast, that bosom is generally most painful which was before affected, and there will be an increased hardness about it, which may give rise, perhaps, to the apprehension of an abscess again forming, or, what is much worse, to the disease terminating in cancer. Both these fears are groundless: and, if she will only use fomentations, gentle friction frequently during the day, with almond oil and laudanum—about a drachm of the latter, to an ounce of the oil, warm,—and exercise patience, everything will do very well.

Nature often seeks her own cure, and a colourless, thin fluid runs from the nipple, which relieves the symptoms.

Cramp, and Pains in the Legs, &c.

Some females, during the latter months of pregnancy, suffer dreadfully from cramp and pain in the legs, and about the sides and lower part of the stomach. This symptom arises from the pressure of the womb upon certain nerves in its neighbourhood, which proceed to the extremities.

If the cramp be seated in the muscles of the legs, a hard, knotty induration is perceivable to the touch, accompanied with great soreness, the latter continuing for a long time after the lump has disappeared. An uneasy position of the muscles is a sufficient cause of irritation, to produce it, and it is frequently removed, by simply rising from the bed or sofa, and walking the room, so as to put the muscles of the leg into action. If this does not succeed, warm friction with the naked hand, or with camphorated oil, generally will.

If spasm affect the sides, or lower part of the stomach, the speediest relief will be obtained from twenty, to five-and-twenty, or thirty drops of laudanum, with a little ether, in distilled peppermint water, or, even at the moment, a little brandy and water; but I generally order, for patients who are at all subject to this affection, the following mixture:—Batley's sedative solution of opium, one drachm; compound tincture of lavender, half an ounce; distilled peppermint water, six ounces. Two tablespoonfuls to be taken before retiring to rest, if there is the slightest intimation of an approaching attack, and also direct that the feet be put into a mustard foot-bath. During the attack, great benefit will be derived from the external application of hot flannels, moistened with the compound camphor liniment.

Violent movements of the Child.

Before the third month of pregnancy, the child is not sufficiently developed to enable it to move. When a little further advanced in growth, it moves, but so feebly and imperfectly, that the mother is not yet sensible of it. A period, however, soon arrives, when its movements, although at first like the mere fluttering of a bird, acquire a power and force, that enable it to give decided proof of life. It is instantly recognised, the female knows she has quickened, and perhaps the sensation experienced is so sudden, that she faints. After this time the motions of the child increase both in frequency and degree, and are readily perceived by the mother, but after a time the womb accustomed to this action within itself, is less sensible of its effects, and except as a satisfactory evidence of the life of the child, is little regarded.

Sometimes, however, the child is *disagreeably active*, so violent as not merely to alarm the mother, but occasion much sickness and uneasiness;—sleepless nights; feverish symptoms, &c., and all this to such an extent, as to require medical interference. If this is not thought necessary, relief will be obtained from losing blood, when not otherwise objectionable, to the amount of a few ounces; gentle aperients, and a night draught containing from twenty-five to thirty drops of Batley's sedative solution of opium. These remedies will afford the greatest relief, and if the symptoms are not altogether removed by them, the female must then endure patiently, recollecting they are a proof that the child is alive and vigorous.*

Soreness and Cracking of the Skin of the Abdomen.

It will sometimes happen during the latter months of pregnancy, that the skin covering the abdomen will not yield readily. This produces much uneasiness; the skin becomes tender and fretted, and if there is very great distension, cracks. It forms a source of great discomfort, and renders the female miserable whenever she moves.

* In many parts of New England, the moccasin root is much used to allay the motions of the child. One tumblerful of the infusion of this root is the usual quantity

It is to be relieved by fomenting the parts with a decoction of poppy-heads;* and the frequent use of warm almond oil, applying in the intervals spermaceti ointment, spread very thinly on a piece of soft linen.

Inconvenience from Size.

Many women in the latter months of gestation experience considerable annoyance, and sometimes severe suffering from the great size of the abdomen, and from want of support, when even not so very large. This is a rare occurrence in a first pregnancy, owing to the firmness of the abdominal muscles, but very frequent in subsequent ones. Little women especially suffer from this unpleasant cause, and, in fact, it is so universally the case with all, who have borne children *rapidly*, that it is highly important for a female to be provided with the means of relieving it.

There is but one remedy with which I am acquainted, but have usually found it answer every purpose. It is wearing during the day-time *a well-applied belt*, next the skin. It must be sufficiently broad for its upper edge to surround the abdomen above the point of its greatest diameter, and its lower

* This decoction is made by taking four ounces of poppy-heads, breaking them up, putting them into a vessel, pouring upon them four pints of boiling water, boiling the whole for fifteen minutes, and then straining off the liquor

edge to come down to, and be supported by, the hips. It must be drawn tight by a lace-string behind, as circumstances may require, and it must likewise be supported by broad straps passing over the shoulders. This will give the required support to the womb, and when the patient is in an upright position, as much as possible of the weight, of what she externally carries, will be thrown upon, or hang from, her shoulders.

Those who suffer much from this cause, ought also to lie down upon a couch or bed for two or three hours every day; this will give great relief to the muscles.

Being Unwell during Pregnancy

A female may be pregnant, and yet be unwell for one period or more while in that condition. Indeed, it may take place every month to the time of quickening, and has even continued in some rare cases up to the time of delivery.

Now, although this can scarcely be called one of the diseases of pregnancy—for it, ordinarily, in no way, interferes with the health—still, as while the discharge is actually present it predisposes to miscarriage, it is necessary to give one or two hints of caution.

Any female, then, thus circumstanced should manage herself with great care immediately before the appearance, during the existence—and directly after the cessation of the discharge. She should observe the most perfect quiet of body and mind—keeping upon the sofa while it lasts, and carefully abstaining from any stimulating or indigestible article of food, and if any symptoms of pain, uneasiness, or threatening miscarriage come on, immediately seek medical advice.

A case, showing the necessity of carefulness under such circumstances, occurred to me some time since, and its relation is all that I need add upon this point.

A lady, resident in Gloucestershire, missing one period, suspected herself of being pregnant, but being unwell on the following month, supposed herself mistaken. She had occasion, however, to come to London on the second day of her being unwell—Monday. On the Wednesday following she suffered considerable uneasiness from the exertion attendant upon the journey, and on Friday while from her hotel was obliged to return home in haste, and before night, miscarried.

Here then is a case in point—first proving, what some persons deny, that a female may be unwell and yet be pregnant, for she could not perceive the slightest difference in the appearance of the discharge from what ordinarily took place, and it was exact as to the time of its return—and next, showing how necessary is great caution, and the most perfect quiet, since undoubtedly this lady would not have miscarried, if her journey had only been delayed another week.

Jaundice sometimes occurs in the early or latter parts of the pregnancy—certain affections also of disordered functions of the heart, producing palpitation—a troublesome cough, accompanied with considerable pain in the head, sudden attacks of difficulty of breathing, and distressing inconvenience from irritable bladder.

These, and many other slight affections, may manifest themselves during gestation, but of those I say nothing. It would be advancing beyond the bounds by which I thought it right to limit myself, and departing from the object proposed.*

* There are one or two complaints to which the pregnant female is subject, upon which a few remarks seem advisable. Speaking of headache, Mr. Fox remarks:—

"Headache, independent of accidents, may be a sympathetic affection arising from disorders of the digestive, or other organs. It may be the consequence of a feeble, or disturbed state of the nervous system: or it may be the effect of the vessels of the head being distended with too much blood; or even of a deficiency of blood in the head.

"Where headache arises from a disordered condition of the digestive organs there will generally be an inactive, or irritable, state of the stomach or bowels, which will frequently be accompanied by giddiness, imperfect vision, or by specks floating a short distance from the eyes, by loss of appetite, sickness, acidity of the contents of the stomach, and by flatulence

"If the stomach be loaded with undigested, or irritating food, it is to be relieved by a gentle emetic. Having drunk a pint of warm chamomile tea, or common tea from one ounce to one ounce and a half of ipecacuanha

I have finished what was purposed, and presented the married female with that in-

wine should be taken, after which vomiting will ensue almost immediately, and without any straining, or painful effort. If ipecacuanha wine is not at hand, two or three teaspoonfuls of powdered mustard, mixed in a little water, may be used in its stead.

"In almost every case, it will be found necessary to administer mild aperients every four or five hours, till the bowels are emptied. The aperients may be, rhubarb and Castile soap, of each one drachm, oil of cloves six drops, mixed with a simple syrup, and divided into thirty pills, of which from three to six are to be taken every four or five hours, till the bowels act. Where no disposition to piles exists, from one to two table spoonfuls of compound decoction of aloes may be taken every four or five hours, till the bowels are relieved freely Where much acidity in the stomach is present, from fifteen to twenty grains of magnesia, combined with six grains of powdered rhubarb, and the same quantity of ginger, may be substituted for the above aperients, and repeated in a similar manner.

"If the pain in the head continues to be severe, after an emetic has operated, or before the aperients begin to act, it will be often greatly mitigated by taking a moderate dose of some opiate; this, however, should not be employed where attacks are frequent, as a habit of taking opiates is productive of much injury.

"There are persons who do not experience relief from opiates, but on the contrary, have the pain aggravated by their use. Strong green tea, or hop tea, will occasionally give relief in mild attacks, or where decided opiates are not productive of benefit.

"Where a feeble, or disturbed state of the nervous system gives rise to headache, aperients are to be taken as recommended above; and stimulants are to be employed, as camphor, ammonia, compound tincture of valerian; æther, &c.

"Four grains of carbonate of ammonia, or fifteen or twenty drops of spirit of hartshorn, are to be mixed in a wineglassful of camphor julep.

"One or two teaspoonfuls of compound tincture of

formation for direction and relief in those little ailments and discomforts which fre

valerian are to be added to a wineglassful of water, or camphor julep.

"From twenty to forty drops of æther are to be mixed in a wineglassful of water or camphor julep.

"Any of the foregoing forms may be taken several times during every twenty-four hours, if necessary.

"If the head is hot, linen wet with vinegar and water, or eau de Cologne and water, is to be repeatedly applied to the temples and forehead; or those parts may be occasionally moistened with æther, the evaporation of which will cause the head to become cool.

"Where reducing the temperature of the head does not diminish the pain, it will be well to try the effect of heat, which may be accomplished in the following manner: pour a little æther into the palm of the hand, and apply it to the forehead, or temples. The heat will be kept up so long as the hand is pressed to the part, and any of the æther remains.

"In severe cases of headache, the patient is to lie perfectly quiet, with the head moderately raised by pillows, and the room is to be darkened.

"If the feet are cold, they should be put into warm water; and if they have a disposition to become chilled again soon, they are to be kept warm by heated flannels, or bottles filled with hot water.

"During an attack of headache, arising from disordered digestive organs, it is essential that the food be very simple, and small in quantity.

"In headache, from nervous disorders, requiring stimulants, the food may be of a nutritious quality; the quantity, however, should be moderate.

"The foregoing remarks apply to sudden, or severe attacks of headache. When slighter affections of the same nature often occur, strict attention to diet, exercise, and the use of aperients, as recommended in a previous chapter, will greatly tend to mitigate the suffering, and to keep off the complaint altogether.

"Where headache comes on in consequence of fulness of the blood-vessels of the head, it will be indicated by quently arise during pregnancy, for which she does not think it necessary to consult her

a sense of weight within the skull, drowsiness, giddiness, particularly on stooping, sickness, ringing or other sounds in the ears, and bright flashes, or sparks in the eyes. In these cases, it will generally be necessary to bleed the temples with eight or ten leeches; and if their application to those parts is known to produce swelling of the eyes and face, the leeches may be placed behind the ears. The head is then to be kept cool by applying cold vinegar and water to it; and purgatives are to be administered.

"The diet is to be very simple, animal food is to be avoided, and no stimulants are to be taken.

"Headache may arise from whatever induces debility It is generally experienced where great loss of blood has taken place, and it may seem singular that the symptoms and sensations of this kind of headache, appear to be the consequence of the vessels of the head having too much blood in them. For instance, there are usually noises resembling the violent beating of a hammer, the rushing of water, the blowing of wind, ringing, &c. It is therefore necessary to notice the condition of the system, to be enabled to decide whether the pain arises from a deficiency, or from an over supply of blood to the head.

"A correct decision should be formed upon this point, by ascertaining whether there is a disposition to fulness of the system, or a state of emptiness of the vessels from great loss of blood, with general debility.

"In the latter case, quietness is most essential: wine and other stimulants, will be necessary; together with a light nutritious diet.

"Opiates also will generally be found requisite, such as have been previously enumerated in this chapter.

"In all cases of headache, mental tranquillity is of much importance; and the patient should not persevere in the pursuit of any occupation which materially increases the pain.

"In this disorder, as well as in many others, accompanied by much irritability, the sleep is often seriously interrupted by slight noises; in most cases, this may be medical adviser, and yet from which she will

prevented by stopping the ears with small plugs, three quarters of an inch in length, and about one quarter of an inch in diameter. If the plugs be made of white wax, they will generally answer the best, as they admit of being accurately moulded to the form of the openings of the ears. Plugs made of turned wood will sometimes be sufficient.

"If such plans as the foregoing do not soon give relief, medical advice should be had, especially where it is supposed that there is too much blood in the vessels of the head.

"Tenderness and irritability of the external parts sometimes come on to an almost intolerable extent, in consequence of inflammatory action. They are most effectually relieved by bathing the parts occasionally with cold or hot water, or decoction of poppy heads, or of laurel leaves, and by using a soothing lotion. The soothing lotion may be made of two drachms of acetate of lead, commonly called sugar of lead, and an ounce of laudanum, in seven ounces of water. It may be applied three or four times during every twenty-four hours.

"In these troublesome affections the bowels must be kept rather more active than usual by gentle aperients. The aperients to be, from two to four drachms of Epsom salts. From one to two teaspoonfuls of electuary of senna. From one to two spoonfuls of castor oil. Or from fifteen to thirty grains of magnesia. Any of which may be taken every second night, or every night, as circumstances may require. The diet should be mild, and there must be a total abstinence from spirit, wine, and malt liquor. If these means fail to give the desired relief, it will be advisable to bleed the parts occasionally with six or eight leeches, and to apply poultices of the same kind, and in the same manner, as recommended in another chapter.

"A discharge frequently appears from the passage, which is either white, or slightly tinged with green, or blood; in such cases, the parts are to be washed, or the passage injected with a syringe, twice daily, with tepid milk and water, or a weak solution of alum in water. For the wash or injection, twelve grains of alum may not unfrequently go on suffering for weeks, rather than speak of them.

be dissolved in six ounces of water, and about two table spoonfuls injected at each time.

"Means should be used to secure the regular action of the bowels, by employing mild aperients and injections, as previously recommended

"More vigorous measures than the above might be productive of much mischief."

PREVENTION TO CONCEPTION.

WE have seen from the preceding pages that in addition to what may be termed diseases ordinarily attendant upon a state of pregnancy, there are others in which to become pregnant is to hazard the health, and often the life of the woman, involving a peremptory necessity either for instrumental or Cæsarean operation, premature delivery or miscarriage. Apart from its agonizing torture, the danger of the Cæsarean operation is imminent to a frightful extent. Premature delivery is often attended with success, but the offspring being prematurely born, if they survive, rarely attain maturity, and even then mostly during their short existence very sickly. Miscarriage, although attended with but little danger when skilfully effected and properly conducted, can only be considered as an alternative; only a choice of evils. But thanks to the indefatigable researches of he learned and humane M.M. Desomeaux or his great discovery by which *pregnancy can be prevented.* By this discovery every woman can have in her own power the means of prevention.

The imperative, and self-evident necessity

that, in some cases, pregnancy should not take place, cannot, for a moment, be doubted, in view that it is within the knowledge of every medical man, who makes his profession subserve the amelioration of the suffering to which the female is subject—knowledge, too, acquired within the sphere of his daily practice—that there are women who should not become pregnant, for with them pregnancy is peril to life. And even when life is spared, the birth of every child snatches many years from the life of the mother, hurrying her, with a constitution shattered, and health destroyed, to a premature grave.

Some women are so constituted that they cannot give birth, not to say to *healthy*, but not to *living* children. Others again cannot give birth at all, except through the instrumental mangling and cutting of the Cæsarean operation—of a piece-meal extraction of the infant from the mother's womb—happy, indeed, if the woman's life fall not a sacrifice to the butchery. Truly, such spectacles are too horrid to contemplate. And yet such women are permitted to become pregnant, in total ignorance that pregnancy ought and can be *prevented*, by safe, simple, invariably healthy, and infallibly certain means.

Some women, again, although not in immediate danger from becoming too frequently pregnant, yet during seven or eight of the nine months of pregnancy, experience the utmost agony of mind and body, making existence a continuous state of misery and suffering, destructive alike of their health, beauty, vigor, and spirits; who, after confinement and recovery, live in constant and perpetual fear and dread of again becoming pregnant, again to undergo the series of intense sufferings from which they have but just emerged. Life, under such circumstances, to the fond and affectionate wife, is but a constant suffering. Can it be otherwise to the kind husband? Can he behold the partner of his joys and sorrows—his bosom companion—the mother of his children—his solace in sickness or difficulty, thus dragging out her days of wretchedness and anguish, emaciated, disheartened, broken in body and spirits; and that, too, in the meridian of her life, in the hey-day of her existence, perceptibly sinking into an early grave, to leave her offspring motherless, or entrust them to the cold and sordid care of the world! Can a husband, possessing the feelings of a man, behold this with indifference; nay, will he not shudder at the possibility of such consequences arising from too frequent pregnancy! Will he not pause and reflect ere he becomes the cause from which such dreadful effects would flow? Surely, if he is a thinking, reflecting, rational, humane man, he must reflect—he must pause, and permit the adoption of the mode pointed out in these pages, by which pregnancy can be prevented, and that, too, without the least sacrifice of those pleasurable sensations experienced in the connubial embrace.

The happiness as well of husband, of wife, and children, will be enhanced by the preservation of her health, by lengthening the intervals between the periods of pregnancy, making the interval between the births three, four, or more years (as in France), depending upon the health of the wife. Thereby it will, under ordinary circumstances, be preserved to rear, guard, and educate her children,—to soothe and comfort the declining years of the father when age and decrepitude are upon him. When, perchance, his own sufferings can be assuaged by only her hand, who alone knows and anticipates his every wish—whose affectionate attention, having accompanied him through the rugged path of life, alone knows how to impart content and happiness.

Surely, then, circumstances do arise where it is folly, madness, wickedness, to permit pregnancy to take place.

Where, for example, the health of the wife evidently sinks under a too frequent state of pregnancy or a too rapid increase of family; or the births taking place in too close succession.

Where the female cannot be in a state of pregnancy without the most intense and excruciating suffering during such period, endangering her own future health, and perhaps that of her offspring.

Where an incapacity exists to give birth

to *living* children, either in consequence of mal-formation of the pelvis, or other deformity; and where, from the same, or other causes, recourse is necessarily had to the Cæsarean operation. All which causes have either the health or the life of the female in view.

But there are still other reasons scarcely less urgent why pregnancy should be sometimes prevented, which have the welfare of the offspring in view.

It is but too lamentable a fact that the sins or misfortunes of the parent are visited upon their offspring. It is indisputable that diseases which carry off their thousands, are, many of them, hereditary,—transmissible from parent to child. Such as confirmed consumption, King's Evil, or Scrofula, Gout, Venereal Disease, Hypochondria, Insanity, and other diseases, and even drunkenness.

In view, then, of the transmission of disease and suffering to our offspring, should they even survive a brief existence, every reflecting being should hesitate whether it were not better to prevent pregnancy than to thrust human beings into the world, and blighting their brief existence with entailed disease and wretchedness—for such offspring are seldom reared to maturity. This fact accounts for the great mortality of children, especially in cities. Those, however, that do pass through a sickly childhood, becoming necessarily endeared to their parents, are cut off in their early years—sometimes in the bloom of youth—blasting the fond hopes just springing into existence in the breasts of their parents. Thus, in some families, five or six, one after another, are apparently prematurely cut off.

The causes, doubtless, to a superficial observer, looking only upon effects, appear inexplicable: not so to those who look beyond mere effects. To such the *present* is but the child of the *past*, and the *parent* of the *future.*

In discussing, therefore, the propriety, the morality, nay, the inevitable necessity, in some cases, of preventing pregnancy, it has an important bearing.

In presenting these considerations, however, we must bear in mind that they are not applicable where the female is capable of enduring the ordinary inconveniences arising from a state of pregnancy, or where her health is not thereby injuriously affected, because the reasons for prevention do not, in such case, exist. Indeed, it is not unusual, that the health of the female, so far from being injured, is often improved, in consequence of the existence of pregnancy, and others, again, who enjoy perfect health without reference to their condition in this respect.

And, again, it is unquestionable that children are often a source of domestic happiness—the binding link—the pledge of affection and love—the delight and joy of parents, upon whose growth and development they look with pride mingled with fond anticipations of the future. The paths of life are made less rugged, the charms of home more pleasant, toil itself becomes less irksome by their influence.

When, therefore, neither the life nor health of the mother is jeopardized, and the offspring free from hereditary or constitutional taint, it is, of course, unnecessary that preventive measures should be used. Neither is it, under such circumstances, recommended.

In regard, however, to the prevention of pregnancy there are still other views, taking still other grounds, treating the subject in a moral and social point of view, which, although not strictly belonging to its consideration in a medical and physiological character, are yet of sufficient interest to be embraced in this work.

The following remarks are from a celebrated physiological writer, and are certainly worthy of consideration, whether we coincide with the author or not. He thus eloquently introduces the subject

"Libertines and debauchees! these pages are not for you. You have nothing to do with the subject of which they treat. Bringing to its discussion, as you do, a distrust or contempt of the human race—accustomed as you are to confound liberty with license, and pleasure with debauchery, it is not for your palled feelings and brutalized senses to distinguish moral truth in its purity and simplicity. I never discuss this subject with such as you.

"It has been remarked, that nothing is so uspicious in a woman, as vehement pretensions to especial chastity; it is no less true, that the most obtrusive and sensitive stickler for the etiquette of orthodox morality is the heartless rake. The little intercourse I have had with men of your stamp, warns me to avoid the serious discussion of any species of moral heresy with you. You approach the subject in a tone and spirit revolting alike to good taste and good feeling. You seem to pre-suppose—from your own experience, perhaps—that the hearts of all men and more especially of all women, are deceitful above all things and desperately wicked; that violence and vice are inherent in human nature, and that nothing but laws and ceremonies prevent the world from becoming a vast slaughter-house, or an universal brothel. You judge your own sex and the other by the specimens you have met with in wretched haunts of mercenary profligacy; and, with such a standard in your minds, I marvel not that you remain incorrigible unbelievers in any virtue, but that which is forced on the prudish hot-bed of ceremonious orthodoxy. I wonder not that you will not trust the natural soil watered from the free skies and warmed by the life-bringing sun. How should you? you have never seen it produce but weeds and poisons. Libertines and debauchees! cast these pages aside! You will find in them nothing to gratify a licentious curiosity; and, if you read them, you will probably only give me credit for motives and impulses like your own.

"And you, prudes and hypocrites! you who strain at a gnat and swallow a camel; you whom Jesus likened to whited sepulchres, which without indeed are beautiful, but within are full of all uncleanness; you who affect to blush if the ankle is incidentally mentioned in conversation, or displayed in crossing a stile, but will read indecencies enough, without scruple, in your closets; you who, at dinner, ask to be helped to the bosom of a duck, lest by mention of the word breast, you call up improper associations; you who have nothing but a head and feet and fingers; you who look demure by daylight, and make appointments only in the dark—you, prudes and hypocrites! I do not address. Even if honest in your prudery, your ideas of right and wrong are too artificial and confused to profit by the present discussion; if dishonest, I desire to have no communication with you.

"Reader! if you belong to the class of prudes or of libertines, I pray you, follow my argument no further. Stop here, and believe that my heresies will not suit you. As a prude, you would find them too honest; as a libertine, too temperate. In the former case, you might call me a very shocking person; in the latter, a quiz or a bore.

"But if you be honest, upright, pure-minded—if you be unconscious of unworthy motive or selfish passion—if truth be your ambition, and the welfare of our race your object—then approach with me a subject the most important to man's well-being; and approach it as I do, in a spirit of dispassionate, disinterested free inquiry. Approach it, resolving to prove all things, and hold fast that which is good. The discussion is one to which it is every man's and every woman's *duty* (and ought to be every one's *business*) to attend. The welfare of the present generation, and—yet far more—of the next, requires it. Common sense sanctions it. And the national motto of my former country, 'Honi soit qui mal y pense,'* may explain the spirit in which it is undertaken, and in which it ought to be received."

* One of the English kings, Edward III., in the year 1344, picked up from the floor of a ball-room, an embroidered garter, belonging to a lady of rank. In returning it to her, he checked the rising smile of his courtiers with the words, "Honi soit qui mal y pense!" or, paraphrased in English, "Shame on him who invidiously interprets it!" The sentiment was so greatly approved, that it has become the motto of the English national arms. It is one which might be not inaptly nor unfrequently applied in rebuking the mawkish, skin-deep, and intolerant morality of this hypocritical and profligate age

PREVENTION TO CONCEPTION;

CONSIDERED

IN ITS SOCIAL BEARINGS.

"What would be the probable effect, in social life, if mankind obtained and exercised a control over the instinct of reproduction?

"My settled conviction is—and I am prepared to defend it—that the effect would be salutary, moral, civilizing; that it would prevent many crimes and more unhappiness; that it would lessen intemperance and profligacy; that it would polish the manners and improve the moral feelings; that it would relieve the burden of the poor, and the cares of the rich; that it would most essentially benefit the rising generation, by enabling parents generally more carefully to educate, and more comfortably to provide for, their offspring. I proceed to substantiate as I may these positions.

"And first, let us look solely to the situation of married persons. Is it not notorious, that the families of the married often increase beyond what a regard for the young beings coming into the world, or the happiness of those who give them birth, would dictate? In how many instances does the hard-working father and more especially the mother of a poor family, remain slaves throughout their lives, tugging at the oar of incessant labor, toiling to live, and living but to toil; when if their offspring had been limited to two or three only, they might have enjoyed comfort and comparative affluence! How often is the health of the mother, giving birth every year to an infant—happy if it be not twins!—and compelled to toil on, even at those times when nature imperiously calls for some relief from daily drudgery—how often is the mother's comfort, health, nay, her life, thus sacrificed! Or, if care and toil have weighed down the spirit, and at last broken the health of the father, how often is the widow left, unable, with the most virtuous intentions, to save her fatherless offspring from becoming degraded objects of charity, or profligate votaries of vice!

"Fathers and mothers! not you who have your nursery and your nursery-maids, and who leave your children at home, to frequent the crowded rout, or to glitter in the hot ball-room; but you by the labor of whose hands your children are to live, and who, as you count their rising numbers, sigh to think how soon sickness or misfortune may lessen those wages which are now but just sufficient to afford them bread—fathers and mothers in humble life! to you my argument comes home, with the force of reality. Others may impugn—may ridicule it. By bitter experience you know and feel its truth

"Yet this is not all. Every physician knows, that there are many women so constituted that they cannot give birth to healthy—sometimes not to *living* children. Is it desirable—is it *moral*, that such women should become pregnant? Yet this is continually the case, the warnings of physicians to the contrary notwithstanding. Others there are, who ought never to become parents; because, if they do, it is only to transmit to their offspring grievous hereditary diseases; perhaps that worst of diseases, insanity. Yet they will not lead a life of celibacy. They marry. They become parents, and the world suffers by it. That a human being should give birth to a child, knowing that he transmits to it hereditary disease, is in my opinion an immorality. But it is a folly to expect that we can ever induce all such persons to live the lives of Shakers. Nor is it necessary; all that duty requires of them is, to refrain from becoming parents. Who can estimate the beneficial effect which rational moral restraint may thus have, on the health, beauty, and physical improvement of our race, throughout future generations?

"But, apart from these latter considerations, is it not most plainly, clearly, incontrovertibly *desirable*, that parents *should have the power** to limit their offspring, whether

* It may perhaps be argued, that all married persons have this power already, seeing that they are no more obliged to become parents than the unmarried; they may

they choose to exercise it or not? Who *can* lose by their having this power? and how many *may* gain! may gain competency for themselves, and the opportunity carefully to educate and provide for their children! How many may escape the jarrings, the quarrels the disorder, the anxiety, which an overgrown family too often causes in the domestic circle?

"It sometimes happens, that individual instances come home to the feelings with greater force than any general reasoning. I shall, in this place, adduce one which came immediately under my cognizance

"In June, 1829, I received from an elderly gentleman of the first respectability, occupying a public situation in one of the western states, a letter requesting to know whether I could afford any information or advice in a case which greatly interested him, and which regarded a young woman for whom he had ever experienced the sentiments of a father. In explanation of the circumstances to which he alluded, he enclosed me a copy of a letter which she had just written to him, and which I here transcribe verbatim. A letter more touching from its simplicity, or more strikingly illustrative of the unfortunate situation in

live as the brethren and sisters among the Shakers do. But this Shaker remedy is, in the first place, utterly impracticable, as a general rule; and, secondly, it would chill and embitter domestic life, even if it were practicable which not one, but thousands, in married life find themselves placed, I have never read.

"'*L*** Kentucky, May* 3, 1829.

"'Dear Sir,

"'The friendship which has existed between you and my father, ever since I can remember; the unaffected kindness you used to express towards me, when you resided in our neighborhood, during my childhood; the lively solicitude you have always seemed to feel for my welfare, and your benevolence and liberal character, induce me to lay before you in a few words, my critical situation, and ask you for your kind advice.

"'It is my lot to be united in wedlock to a young mechanic of industrious habits, good dispositions, pleasing manners, and agreeable features, excessively fond of our children and of me; in short, eminently well qualified to render himself and family and all around him happy, were it not for the besetting sin of drunkenness. About once in every three or four weeks, if he meet, either accidentally or purposely, with some of his friends, of whom, either real or pretended his good nature and liberality procure him many, he is sure to get intoxicated, so as to lose his reason; and, when thus beside himself, he trades and makes foolish bargains, so much to his disadvantage, that he has almost reduced himself and family to beggary, be-

ing no longer able to keep a shop of his own, but obliged to work journey work.

"'We have not been married quite four years, and have already given being to three dear little ones. Under present circumstances, what can I expect will be their fate and mine? I shudder at the prospect before me. With my excellent constitution and industry, and the labor of my husband, I feel able to bring up these three little cherubs in decency, were I to have no more: but when I seriously consider my situation, I can see no other alternative left for me, than to tear myself away from the man who, though addicted to occasional intoxication, would sacrifice his life for my sake; and for whom, contrary to my father's will, I successively refused the hand and wealth of a lawyer and of a preacher; or continue to witness his degradation, and bring into existence, in all probability, a numerous family of helpless and destitute children, who, on account of poverty, must inevitably be doomed to a life of ignorance, and consequent vice and misery.

"'M. W.'"

"Need I add one word of comment on such a case as this? Every feeling mind must be touched by the amiable feeling and good sense that pervade the letter. Every rational being, surely, must admit, that the power of preventing, without injury or sacrifice, the increase of a family, under such circumstances, is a public benefit and a private blessing.

"Will it be asserted—and I know no other even plausible reply to these facts and arguments—will it be asserted, that the thing is, in itself, immoral or unseemly? I deny it; and I point to the population of France, in justification of my denial. Where will you find, on the face of the globe, a more polished or more civilized nation than the French, or one more punctiliously alive to any rudeness, coarseness or indecorum? You will find none. The French are scrupulous on these points, to a proverb. Yet, as every intelligent traveller in France must have remarked, there is scarcely to be found, among the middle or upper classes (and seldom even among the working classes), such a thing as a large family; very seldom more than three or four children. A French lady of the utmost delicacy and respectability will, in common conversation, say as simply —(ay, and as *innocently*, whatever the self-righteous prude may aver to the contrary)—as she would proffer any common remark about the weather: "'I have three children; my husband and I think that is as many as we can do justice to, and I do not intend to have any more.'"*

* Will our sensitive fine ladies blush at the plain good sense and simplicity of such an observation? Let me tell them, the indelicacy is in their own minds, not in the words of the French mother

"I have stated notorious facts, facts which no traveller who has visited Paris, and seen anything of the domestic life of its inhabitants, will attempt to deny. However heterodox, then, my view of the subject may be in this country, I am supported in it by the opinion and the practice of the most refined and most socially cultivated nation in the world.

"Will it still be argued, that the practice, if not coarse, is immoral? Again, I appeal to France. I appeal to the details of the late glorious revolution—to the innumerable instances of moderation, of courage, of honesty, of disinterestedness, of generosity, of magnanimity, displayed on the memorable 'three days,' and ever since; and I challenge comparison between the national character of France for virtue, as well as politeness, and that of any other nation under heaven.

"It is evident, then, that to married persons, the power of limiting their offspring to their circumstances is most desirable. It may often promote the harmony, peace, and comfort of families; sometimes it may save from bankruptcy and ruin, and sometimes it may rescue the mother from premature death. In *no* case can it, by possibility, be worse than superfluous. In *no case can it be mischievous.*

"If the moral feelings were carefully cultivated, if we were taught to consult, in everything, rather the welfare of those w love than our own, how strongly would these arguments be felt? No man ought even to *desire* that a woman should become the mother of his children, unless it was her express wish, and unless he knew it to be for her welfare, that she should. Her feelings, her interests, should be for him in this matter *an imperative law.* She it is who bears the burden, and therefore with her also should the decision rest. Surely it may well be a question whether it be desirable, or whether any man ought to ask, that the whole life of an intellectual, cultivated woman, should be spent in bearing a family of twelve or fifteen children; to the ruin, perhaps, of her constitution, if not to the overstocking of the world. No man ought to require or expect it.

"Shall I be told, that this is the very romance of morality? Alas that what ought to be a matter of every-day practice—a commonplace exercise of the duties and charities of life—a bounden duty—an instance of domestic courtesy too universal either to excite remark or to merit commendation—alas! that a virtue so humble that its absence ought to be reproached as a crime, should, to our selfish perceptions, seem but a fastidious refinement, or a fanciful supererogation!

"But I pass from the case of married persons to that of young men and women who have yet formed no matrimonial connexion.

" In the present state of the world, when public opinion stamps with opprobrium every sexual connection which has not received the orthodox sanction of an oath, almost all young persons, on reaching the age of maturity, desire to marry. The heart must be very cold, or very isolated, that does not find some object on which to bestow its affections. Thus, early marriages would be almost universal, did not prudential considerations interfere. The young man thinks, 'I must not marry yet. I cannot support a family. I must make money first, and think of a matrimonial settlement afterwards.'

" And so he goes to making money, fully and sincerely resolved, in a few years to share it with her whom he now loves. But passions are strong, and temptations great. Curiosity, perhaps, introduces him into the company of those poor creatures whom society first reduces to a dependence on the most miserable of mercenary trades, and then curses for being what she has made them. There his health and his moral feelings alike are made shipwreck. The affections he had thought to treasure up for their first object, are chilled by dissipation and blunted by excess. He scarcely retains a passion but avarice. Years pass on—years of profligacy and speculation—and his first wish is accomplished; his fortune is made. Where now are the feelings and resolves of his youth

"'Like the dew on the mountain,
Like the foam on the river,
Like the bubble on the fountain,
They are gone—and for ever?'

"He is a man of pleasure—a man of the world. He laughs at the romance of his youth, and marries a fortune. If gaudy equipages and gay parties confer happiness, he is happy. But if these be only the sunshine on the stormy ocean below, he is a victim to that system of morality which forbids a reputable connexion until the period when provision has been made for a large, expected family. Had he married the first object of his choice, and simply delayed becoming a father until his prospects seemed to warrant it, how different might have been his lot! Until men and women are absolved from the fear of becoming parents, except when they themselves desire it, they ever will form mercenary and demoralizing connexions, and seek in dissipation the happiness they might have found in domestic life.

"I know that this, however common, is not an universal case. Sometimes the heavy responsibilities of a family are incurred at all risks; and who shall say how often a life of unremitting toil and poverty is the consequence? Sometimes—if even rarely—the young mind *does* hold to its first resolves. The youth plods through years of cold celibacy and solitary anxiety; happy, if before the best hours of life are gone, and its warmest feelings withered, he may return to claim the reward of his forbearance and of his industry. But even in this comparatively happy case, shall we count for nothing the years of ascetical sacrifice at which after-happiness is purchased? The days of youth are not too many, nor its affections too lasting. We may, indeed, if a great object require it, sacrifice the one and mortify the other. But is this, in itself, desirable? Does not wisdom tell that such sacrifice is a dead loss—to the warm-hearted often a grievous one? Does not wisdom bid us temperately enjoy the spring-time of life, 'while the evil days come not, nor the years draw nigh' when we shall say, 'we have no pleasure in them?'

"Let us say, then, if we will, that the youth who thus sacrifices the present for the future, chooses wisely between two evils, profligacy and asceticism. This is true. But let us not imagine the lesser evil to be a good. It is *not* good for man to be alone. It is for no man's or woman's happiness or benefit that they should be condemned to Shakerism. It is a violence done to the feelings, and an injury to the character. A life of rigid celibacy, though infinitely preferable to a life of dissipation, is yet fraught with many evils. Peevishness, restlessness, vague longings, and instability of character, are among the least of these. The mind is unsettled, and the judgment warped. Even the very instinct which is thus mortified assumes an undue importance, and occupies a portion of the thoughts which does not of right or nature belong to it; and which, during a life of satisfied affection, it would not obtain.

"I speak not now of extreme cases, where solitary vice* or disease, or even insanity, has been the result of ascetical mortification. I speak of every day cases; and I am well convinced that (however wise it often is, in the present state of the world, to select and adhere to this alternative), yet no man or woman can live the life of a conscientious Shaker, without suffering, more or less, both physically, mentally, and morally. This is the more to be regretted, because the very noblest portion of our species—the good, the pure, the high-minded, and the kind-hearted —are the chief victims.

"Thus, inasmuch as the scruple of incur-

* For a vice so unnatural as onanism there could be no possible temptation, and therefore no existence, were not men unnaturally and mischievously situated. It first appeared, probably in monasteries; and has been perpetuated by the more or less anti-social and demoralizing relation in which the sexes stand to each other, in almost all countries. In estimating the consequences of the present false situation of society, we must set down to the black account the wretched consequences (terminating not unfrequently in incurable insanity) of this vice, the preposterous offspring of modern civilization. Physicians say that onanism at present prevails, to a lamentable extent, both in this country and in England. If the recommendations contained in these pages were generally followed, it would probably totally disappear in a single generation

ring heavy responsibilities deters from forming moral connexions, and encourages intemperance and prostitution, the knowledge which enables man to limit his offspring, would, in the present state of things, save much unhappiness and prevent many crimes. Young persons sincerely attached to each other, and who might wish to marry, would marry early; merely resolving not to become parents until prudence permitted it. The young man, instead of solitary toil or vulgar dissipation, would enjoy the society and the assistance of her he had chosen as his companion; and the best years of life, whose pleasures never return, would not be squandered in riot, or lost through mortification.

"My readers will remark, that all the arguments I have hitherto employed, apply strictly to the present order of things, and the present laws and system of marriage. No one, therefore, need be a moral heretic on this subject to admit and approve them. The marriage laws might all remain for ever as they are; and yet a moral check to population would be beneficent and important.

"But there are other cases, it will be said, where the knowledge of a preventive would be mischievous. If young women, it will be argued, were absolved from the fear of consequences, they would rarely preserve their chastity. Unlegalized connexions would be common and seldom detected. Seduction would be facilitated. Let us dispassionately examine this argument.

"I fully agree with that most amiable of moral heretics, Shelley, that 'Seduction, which term could have no meaning in a rational society, has now a most tremendous one.'* It matters not how artificial the penalty which society has chosen to affix to a breach of her capricious decrees. Society has the power in her own hands; and that moral Shylock, Public Opinion, enforces the penalty, even though it cost the life of the victim. The consequences, then, to the poor sufferer, whose offence is, at most, but an error of judgment or a weakness of the heart, are the same as if her imprudence were indeed a crime of the blackest dye. And his conduct who, for a momentary, selfish gratification, will deliberately entail a life of wretchedness on one whose chief fault, perhaps, was her misplaced confidence in a villain, is not one whit excused by the folly and injustice of the sentence.† Some poet says,

* See letter of Percy Bysshe Shelley, published in the "Lion," of December 5, 1828.

† Every reflecting mind will distinguish between the unreasoning—sometimes even generous, imprudence of youthful passion, and the calculating selfishness of the matured and heartless libertine. It is a melancholy truth, that pseudo-civilization produces thousands of seducers by profession, who, while daily calling the heavens to witness their eternal affections, have no affection for anything on earth but their own precious and profligate selves. It is to characters so utterly worthless as these that my observations apply.

> 'The man who lasys his hands upon a woman,
> Save in the way of kindness, is a wretch
> Whom 'twere gross flattery to call a coward.'

What epithet then belongs to him who makes it a trade to win a woman's gentle affections, betray her generous confidence, and then, when the consequences become apparent, abandon her to dependence, and the scorn of a cold, a self-righteous, and a wicked world; a world which will forgive anything but rebellion against its tyranny, and in whose eyes it seems the greatest of crimes to be unsuspecting and warm-hearted! I will give my hand freely to a galley-slave, and speak to the highway-robber as to an honest man; but there is one character with whom I desire to exchange neither word nor greeting—the cold-hearted, deliberate, practised, and calculating seducer!

"And, let me ask, what is it gives to the arts of seduction their sting, and stamps to the world its victim? Why is it, that the man goes free and enters society again, almost courted and applauded for his treachery, while the woman is a mark for the finger of reproach, and a butt for the tongue of scandal? Because she bears about her the mark of what is called her disgrace. She becomes a mother; and society has something tangible against which to direct its anathemas. Nine-tenths, at least, of the misery and ruin which are caused by seduction, even in the present state of public opinion on the subject, result from cases of pregnancy.

"If the little being lives, the dove in the falcon's claws is not more certain of death, than we may be, that society will visit, with its bitterest scoffs and reproaches, the bruised spirit of the mother and the unconscious innocence of the child.

"If, then, we cannot do all, shall we neglect a part? If we cannot prevent every misery which man's selfishness and the world's cruelty entail on a sex which it ought to be our pride and honor to cherish and defend; let us prevent as many as we can. If we cannot persuade society to revoke its unmanly and *unchristian** persecution of those who are often the best and gentlest of its members—let us, at the least, give to woman what defence we may, against its violence.

"I appeal to any father, trembling for the reputation of his child, whether, if she were induced to form an unlegalized connexion, her pregnancy would not be a frightful aggravation? I appeal to him, whether a preventive which shall save her from a situation which must soon disclose all to the world, would not be an act of mercy, of charity, of philanthropy—whether it might not save him from despair, and her from ruin? The fastidious conformist may frown upon the question, but to the father it comes

* Jesus said unto her, "Neither do I condemn thee." *John* viii., 11

home; and, whatever his lips may say, his heart will acknowledge the soundness and the force of the argument it conveys.

"It may be, that sticklers for morality will still demur to the positions I defend. They will perhaps tell me, as the committee of a certain society in this city lately did—that the power of preventing conception 'holds out inducements and facilities for the prostitution of their daughters, their sisters, and their wives.'

"Truly, but they pay their wives, their sisters, and their daughters, a poor compliment! Is, then, this vaunted chastity a mere thing of circumstance and occasion? Is there but the difference of opportunity between it and prostitution? Would their wives, and their sisters, and their daughters, if once absolved from the fear of offspring, all become prostitutes—and sell their embrace for gold, and descend to a level with the most degraded? In truth, but they slander their own kindred: they libel their own wives, sisters, and daughters. If they spoke truth—if fear were indeed the only safeguard of their relatives' chastity, little value should I place on virtue like that! and small would I esteem his offence, who should attempt to seduce it.*

* I should like to hear these gentlemen explain, according to what principle they imagine the chastity of their *wives* to grow out of a fear of offspring; so that, if released from such fear, prostitution would follow. I

"That chastity which is worth preserving is not the chastity that owes its birth to fear and to ignorance. If to enlighten a woman regarding a simple physiological fact will make her a prostitute, she must be especially

can readily comprehend that the unmarried may be supposed carefully to avoid that situation to which no legal cause can be assigned; but a wife must be especially dull, if she cannot assign, in all cases, a legal cause; and a husband must be especially sagacious, if he can tell whether the true cause be assigned or not This safeguard to married chastity, therefore, to which the gentlemen of the Committee alluded to seem to look with so implicit a confidence, is a mere broken reed; and has been so ever since the days of Bethsheba.

Yet *conjugal* chastity is that which is especially valued. The inconstancy of a wife commonly cuts much deeper than the dishonour of a sister. In that case, then, which the world usually considers of the highest importance, the fear of offspring *imposes no check whatever* It cannot make one iota of difference whether a married woman be knowing in physiology or not; except perhaps, indeed, to the husband's advantage; in cases where the wife's conscience induces her at least to guard against the possibility of burthening her legal lord with the care and support of children that are not his. Constancy, where it actually exists, is the offspring of something more efficacious than ignorance. And if in the wife's case, men must and do trust to something else, why not in all other cases, where restraint may be considered desirable? Shall men trust in the greater, and fear to trust in the less? Whatever any one may choose to assert regarding his relatives' secret inclinations to profligacy, these arguments may convince him that if he has any safeguard at present, a perusal of these pages will not destroy it.

'Tis strange that men, by way of suborning an argument, should be willing thus to vilify their relatives' character and motives, without first carefully examining whether anything was gained to their cause, after all, by the vilification.

predisposed to profligacy. But it is a libel on the sex. Few, indeed, there are, who would continue so miserable and degrading a calling, could they but escape from it. For one prostitute that is made by inclination, ten are made by necessity. Reform the laws—equalize the comforts of society, and you need withhold no knowledge from your wives and daughters. It is want, not knowledge, that leads to prostitution.

For myself, I would withhold from no sister, or daughter, or wife of mine, any ascertained fact whatever. It should be to me a duty and a pleasure to communicate to them all I knew myself; and I should hold it an insult to their understandings and their hearts to imagine, that their virtue would diminish as their knowledge increased. Vice is never the offspring of just knowledge, and they who say it is, slander their own nature. Would we but trust human nature, instead of continually suspecting it, and guarding it by bolts and bars, and thinking to make it very chaste by keeping it very ignorant, what a different world we should have of it! The virtue of ignorance is a sickly plant, ever exposed to the caterpillar of corruption, liable to be scorched and blasted even by the free light of heaven; of precarious growth; and even if at last artificially matured, of little or no real value.

"I know that parents often think it right and proper to withhold from their children—

especially from their daughters—facts the most influential on their future lives, and the knowledge of which is essential to every man and woman's well-being.* Such a course has ever appeared to me ill-judged and productive of very injurious effects. A girl is surely no whit the better for believing,

* Instances innumerable might be adduced. Not one young person, for example, in twenty, is ever told, that sexual intercourse during the period of a woman's courses is not unfrequently productive to the woman of a species of fluor albus, and sometimes (as a consequent) to the man of symptoms very similar to those of urethritis or gonorrhœa, but more easily removed. Yet what fact more important to be communicated? And how ridiculous the mischievously prudish refinement that conceals from human beings what it most deeply concerns them to know? The following case is related by Dr. Dewees in his work on Diseases of Females: "We have known a complaint communicated to the male by intercourse with a woman labouring under *Pruritis*. It was very similar to that which affected the female in its general character. When this occurs with the married man, much disturbance is sometimes created from a supposition that the wife has been unfaithful, and the contrary Indeed, it has occurred in more instances than one within our own knowledge, where the woman has thought herself the injured party; and in one case the recrimination was mutual. In this instance, the friends of the parties assembled to determine on the terms of separation, when it was suggested, by one of those who happened to be more rational than the rest, that before they proceeded to such an extremity, their family physician should be consulted. We were accordingly sent for. After an attentive hearing of both parties, and an examination of the parts, we were satisfied that there was not the slightest ground for either to be charged with want of fidelity, and we assured the parties that this was the case, and were fortunate enough to cause all further proceedings to be suspended."

until her marriage night, that children are found among the cabbage leaves in the garden. The imagination is excited, the curiosity kept continually on the stretch; and that which, if simply explained, would have been recollected only as any other physiological phenomenon, assumes all the rank and importance and engrossing interest of a mystery. Nay, I am well convinced, that mere curiosity has often led ignorant young people into situations, from which a little more confidence and openness on the part of their parents and guardians, would have effectually secured them.

"But if we *could* prevent the circulation of truth, why *should* we? We are not afraid of it ourselves. No man thinks *his* morality will suffer by it. Each feels certain that his virtue can stand any degree of knowledge. And is it not the height of egregious presumption in each to imagine that his neighbor is so much weaker than himself, and requires a bandage which he can do without? Most of all is it presumptuous to suppose, that that knowledge which the man of the world can bear with impunity, will corrupt the young and the pure-hearted. It is the sullied conscience only that suggests such fears. Trust youth and innocence. Speak to them openly. Show them that you respect them, by treating them with confidence; and they will quickly learn to respect and to govern themselves. You enlist even their pride in your behalf; and you will soon see them make it their boast and their highest pleasure to *merit* your confidence. But watch them and show your suspicions of them but once, —and you are the jailor, who will keep his prisoners just as long as bars and bolts shall prevent their escape. The world was never made for a prison-house; it is too large and ill-guarded: nor were parents ever intended for jail-keepers; their very affections unfit them for the task.

"There is no more beautiful sight on earth, than a family among whom there are no secrets and no reserves; where the young people confide everything to their elder friends—for such to them are their parents —and where the parents trust everything to their children; where each thought is communicated as freely as it arises; and all knowledge given, as simply as it is received. If the world contain a prototype of that Paradise, where nature is said to have known no sin or impropriety, it is such a family; and if there be a serpent that can poison the innocence of its inmates, that serpent is SUSPICION.

"I ask no greater pleasure than thus to be the guardian and companion of young beings whose innocence shall speak to me as unreservedly as it thinks to itself; of young beings who shall never imagine that there is guilt in their thoughts, or sin in their confidence; and to whom, in return, I may impart every important and useful fact that is known to myself. Their virtue shall be of that hardy growth, which *all* facts tend to nourish and strengthen.

"I put it to my readers, whether such a view of human nature, and such a mode of treating it, be not in accordance with the noblest feelings of their hearts. I put it to them, whether they have not felt themselves encouraged, improved, strengthened in every virtuous resolution, when they were generously trusted; and whether they have not felt abased and degraded, when they were suspiciously watched, and spied after, and kept in ignorance. If they find such feelings in their own hearts, let them not self-righteously imagine, that they can only be won by generosity, or that the nature of their fellow-creatures is different from their own.

"There are other considerations connected with this subject, which farther attest the social advantages of the control I advocate. Human affections are mutable, and the sincerest of moral resolutions may change.* Every day furnishes instances of alienations and of separations; sometimes almost before the honey-moon is well expired. In such

* Le premier serment que se firent deux êtres de chair ce fut au pied d'un rocher, qui tombait en poussiere; il attestèrent de leur constance un ciel qui n'est pas un instant le même: tout passait en eux, et autour d'eux; e ils croyaient leurs cœurs affranchis de vicissitudes. O enfans! toujours enfans.

DIDEROT; *Jacques et son Maitre*

cases of unsuitability, it cannot be considered desirable that there should be offspring; and the power of refraining from becoming parents until intimacy had, in a measure, established the likelihood of permanent harmony of views and feelings, must be confessed to be advantageous.

"It would be impossible to meet every argument in detail, which ingenuity or prejudice might put forward. If the world were not actually afraid to think freely or to listen to the suggestions of common sense, three-fourths of what has already been said would be superfluous; for most of the arguments employed would occur spontaneously to any rational, reasoning being. But the mass of mankind have still, in a measure, everything to learn on this subject. The world seems to me much to resemble a company of gourmands, who sit down to a plentiful repast, first very punctiliously saying grace over it; and then, under the sanction of the priest's blessing, think to gorge themselves with impunity; as conceiving, that gluttony after grace is no sin. So it is with popular customs and popular morality. Everything is permitted, if external forms be but respected. Legal roguery is no crime, and ceremony sanctioned excess no profligacy. The substance is sacrificed to the form, the virtue to the outward observance. The world troubles its head little about whether a man be honest or dishonest, so he knows how to avoid the penitentiary and escape the hangman. In like manner, the world seldom thinks it worth while to inquire whether a man be temperate or intemperate, prudent or thoughtless. It takes especial care to inform itself whether in all things he conforms to orthodox requirements; and if he does, all is right. Thus men too often learn to consider an oath an absolution from all subsequent decencies and duties, and a full release from all responsibilities. If a husband maltreat his wife, the offence is venal; for he premised it by making her at the altar, an 'honest woman.' If a married father neglects his children, it is a trifle; for grace was regularly said before they were born.

"With such a world as this, it is a difficult matter to reason. After listening to all I have said, it may perhaps cut me short by reminding me, that nature herself declares it to be right and proper, that we should reproduce our species without calculation or restraint. I will ask, in reply, whether nature also declares it to be right and proper, that when the thermometer is at 96°, we should drink greedily of cold water, and drop down dead in the streets? Let the world be told, that if nature gave us our passions and propensities, she gave us also the power wisely to control them; and that, when we hesitate to exercise that power we descend to a level with the brute creation, and become the sport of fortune—the mere slaves of circum stance.*

"To one other argument it were not, perhaps, worth while to advert, but that it has been already speciously used to excite popu lar prejudice. It has been said, that to re commend to mankind prudential restraint in cases where children cannot be provided for is an insult to the poor man; since all ought to be so circumstanced that they might pro vide amply for the largest family. Most as suredly all *ought* to be so circumstanced, but all *are* not. And there would be just as much propriety in bidding a poor man to go and take by force a piece of Saxony broad-cloth from his neighbor's store, because he *ought* to be able to purchase it, as to encourage him to go on producing children, because he *ought* to have the wherewithal to support them. Let us exert every nerve to correct the injustice and arrest the misery that re sults from a vicious order of things; but, un til we have done so, let us not, for humanity's sake, madly recommend that which grievous

* Some German poet, whose name has escaped me, says

"Tapfer ist de Lowensieger,
Tapfer is der Weltbezwinger,
Tapferer, wer sich selbst bezwang!"

"Brave is the lion-victor,
Brave the conqueror of a world,
Braver he who controls himself!"

It is a noble sentiment, and very appropriate to the pre sent discussion.

ly aggravates the evil; which increases the burden on the present generation, and threatens with neglect and ignorance the next.

"It now remains, after having spoken of the *desirability* of obtaining control over the instinct of reproduction, to speak of its *practicability*.

"I have taken great pains to ascertain the opinions of the most enlightened physicians of Great Britain and France on this subject; (opinions which popular prejudice will not permit them to offer publicly in their works;) and they all concur in admitting, what the experience of the French nation *positively proves*, that man may have a perfect control over this instinct: and that men and women may, without any injury to health, or the slightest violence done to the moral feelings, and with but small diminution to the pleasure which accompanies the gratification of the instinct, refrain at will from becoming parents. It has chanced to me, also, to win the confidence of several individuals, who have communicated to me, without reserve, their own experience: and all this has been corrobative of the same opinion.

"However various and contradictory the different theories of generation, almost all physiologists are agreed, that the entrance of the sperm itself (or of some volatile particles proceeding from it) into the uterus, must precede conception. This it was that probably first suggested the possibility of preventing conception at all."

The eloquent writer, who was at that time unaware of the existence of Desomeaux's mode of prevention to conception,* states

* The author of these pages having resided many years in France, where this preventive has been used with infallible and invariable success, can vouch for its efficacy, healthiness and certainty. While there, he was importuned to take the agency for its disposal in the United States. But aware of the extreme sensitiveness, verging upon mawkishness, with which the agitation of a question of this nature would be viewed; the misapprehension to which it might give rise, and the difficulty of presenting it to the consideration of the public, it was not without some reluctance that he was induced to take the exclusive agency for its sale in this country. The numerous testimonials, however, of its efficacy, and the warm expressions of gratitude and thankfulness he has received since taking the agency, have convinced him that this invaluable preventive has been appreciated.

Its efficacy is beyond question, as in Europe, among the higher classes especially, it is universally used, and of late among all classes. Thousands of married persons have for years used it with invariable success. Instances are related by the author from whom we have liberally quoted, exactly similar to hundreds which have come to the knowledge of the writer of these pages. The principle upon which it prevents conception, is to neutralize the fecundating properties in semen, and it preserves and conduces to the health of the female, by eradicating all predisposition to sexual weakness, fluor albus, or whites, the falling of the womb, &c., and restores and maintains that elasticity and firmness of the generative functions (appertaining only to a young female) for many years. The French, who are scrupulously observant of themselves in these particulars, and who retain their health, vivacity, and capacity to receive and impart enjoyment, to a remarkable age, would not for worlds abstain from the use of M. Desomeaux's Preventive to Conception, the same result was attained by a complete withdrawal on the part of the male previous to emission. But this mode, it will be readily perceived, is attended with, to some, insurmountable difficulties.

In the first place, few men can invariably control themselves in this respect, and to be an effectual preventive, he must ever, and invariably control his passions. Now it can not be denied, that even those who habitually can, and do control themselves, will inevitably, now and then, in so exciting a passion, lose their self-control. It is impossible to do otherwise. And one moment's forgetfulness defeats the end. In the second place, even if always and invariably practicable, it makes the act of coition incomplete and unsatisfactory. In the third place it would be almost nay quite impossible, to prevent an impercept

merely from its effects in preserving their youth to an old age, and would not permit a sexual act to transpire without its use. When used under these circumstances, the directions are somewhat varied. It is well known that the French always have intervals of three, four, or more years, between the birth of children, depending upon either the health of the wife, or inclination or judgment of parents. In cases of mal-formation, deformity of pelvis, low state of health, its use is indispensable. In obtaining this celebrated preventive, it is advisable in all cases to communicate directly with him, the sole agent of the United States, for the disposal of "*M. Desomeaux's Preventive to Conception.*" The packages can be forwarded to all parts of the United States. Letters must be post-paid, and addressed to Dr. A. M. Mauriceau, Box "1224," N. Y. Office 129 Liberty-street, N. Y. Price of package, Ten Dollars ible and unconscious escape of semen, sufficient however to produce conception, often giving rise to unjust and unfounded suspicions, when, in fact, the cause for the existence of pregnancy is the same as though no withdrawal was practised. And lastly, its effects upon the constitution are frequently not unlike those produced by onanism. In addition to which, it is unsafe, because uncertain; consequently, when indispensable to prevent pregnancy, is of no avail, if not actually dangerous.*

To sum up, in brief, why pregnancy should be prevented, the reasons adduced seem to be conclusive to the able and talented writer, in its moral, social, and physiological aspect.

Morally. Firstly. It induces early marriages by removing the principal obstacle

* In France, and on the Continent of Europe generally, a covering (used by the male), called a *baudruche* (known as the French Secret), is used with success, with the view of preventing pregnancy. Its intention, however, and for which, perhaps, it is specially adapted, is to obviate the penalty incurred by prostitution, and thereby guard against the contraction of syphilis. But as the object of the author is not to facilitate, but, on the contrary, effectually to prevent the degrading intercourse the consequences of which are sought to be avoided, in adverting to it therefore, he has only in view its adaptation to prevent conception. If made of proper material and texture it can, to a certain extent, be relied upon. Deeming this latter consideration of essential importance, and having been applied to in regard to it, he has imported them made of the only material of which they should be composed. Address Dr. A. M. Mauriceau, Box "1224," N. Y. City, who will send them by mail to any part of the United States. Price $5 a dozen.

thereto, viz.: the fear of having offspring before the parents are in a pecuniary condition to support, rear, and educate them. And,

Secondly, By inducing early marriages, seductions would become less frequent, and consequently prostitution, comparatively, become extinct.

Socially. Firstly. Young men, instead of seeking excitement and amusement in the intoxicating cup, gaming, night carousals, brothels, &c., acquiring habits of dissipation deadening alike to the keen, fresh susceptibilities belonging to youth—habits too, which often cling to them in after life, habits which, perhaps for ever destroy their health,—as tainting their constitution with some foul and incurable disease,—would, with a view to early marriage, cultivate the social and domestic ties, while yet pure and uncontaminated by contact with the dissolute and vicious. And

Secondly, Young persons, even though with very limited means, would nevertheless marry, and by not becoming parents, be enabled, unitedly, to husband their resources with the view to the bettering their condition pecuniarily; in the meantime, and in the days of their youth, enjoying all those social endearments which each sex finds in the society of the other, where reciprocity of views, interests, and feelings exists. So too those in middling circumstances would marry early, merely deferring an increase of family until they will have established themselves in some business, ere the constant accumulating expenses of an increasing family encroach upon, or eat up their small capital, he immediate incurrence of which thus early would, perhaps, for ever destroy the means for the comfortable provision of themselves, as also the future welfare of their children.

Physiologically. By inducing early marriages, the dire evils arising from promiscuous sexual intercourse with the tainted or diseased, will gradually disappear, and in a generation or two we would find springing up, in the place of the present sickly, puny race, a healthy, robust, and pure generation.

In regard to the morality of preventing conception it is contended that everything which tends to the amelioration of mankind, to improve their condition physically, morally, and socially, or equalize their condition pecuniarily, cannot be immoral. That the instinct of reproduction should be, like our other appetites and passions, subject to the control of reason,—that when the gratification of this instinct results in evil effects either to ourselves or to our offspring, or even to society—if such evil can be prevented, it is the obligation of morality that it should be.

It is contended, then, that the use of a preventive to conception will make men and women rational, reflecting, thinking beings, regardful alike of their own welfare and the welfare of their offspring. That it will banish poverty, vice and profligacy, by enabling the poor to improve their pecuniary condition and thus engendering habits of frugality, reflection and economy, which the prospect of future competency is so calculated to inspire. Vice so often springing from despair and hopeless poverty will disappear, because the children, by reason of the competence and moral structure of the parents, will not in infancy be thrust upon the world to mingle with the depraved and the licentious. Sexual profligacy and licentiousness will be checked, as early marriages become more prevalent and universal, as there then will exist no reasons as now, why two persons, attached to each other, should not marry, refraining merely from becoming parents. Dishonorable advances therefore would be spurned, seductions thus have no existence, and prostitution, the offspring of seduction, would be unknown, and even the ravages of that disease, engendered by promiscuous sexual intercourse, now carrying off its tens of thousands, transmitting its pestiferous poison to thousands yet unborn, would entirely disappear.

The able author thus concludes his views

"And now let my readers pause. Let them review the various arguments I have placed before them. Let them reflect how intimately the instinct of which I treat is connected with the social welfare of society Let them bear in mind, that just in proportion to its social influence, is it important that we should know how to control and govern t; that when we obtain such control, we may save ourselves—and, what we ought to prize much more highly, may save our companions and our offspring, from suffering or misery; that, by such knowledge, the young may form virtuous connexions, instead of becoming profligates or ascetics; that, by it, early marriage is deprived of its heaviest consequences, and seduction of its sharpest sting; that, by it, man may be saved from moral ruin, and woman from desolating dishonor; that by it the first pure affections may be soothed and satisfied, instead of being thwarted or destroyed—let them call to mind all this, and let them say, whether the possession of such control be not a blessing to man.

"As to the cry which prejudice may raise against it as being unnatural, it is just as unnatural (and no more so) as to refrain, in a sultry summer's day, from drinking, perhaps, more than a pint of water at a draught, which prudence tells us is enough, while inclination would bid us drink a quart. *All* thwarting of any human wish or impulse may, in one sense, be called unnatural; it is not, however, ofttimes the less prudent and proper on that account."

As to the practical efficacy of this preventive, the experience of France, where it is universally practised, might suffice in proof. We know, at this moment, several married persons who have told us, that, after having had as many children as they thought prudent, *they had for years employed it with perfect success.* For the satisfaction of our readers, we will select some instances.

A few weeks since, a respectable and very intelligent father of a family, about thirty-five years of age, who resides west of the mountains, called at our office. Conversation turned on the present subject, and we expressed to him our conviction that this preventive was effectual. He told us he could speak from personal experience. He had married young, and soon had three children. These he could support in comfort, without running into debt or difficulty; but, the price of produce sinking in his neighborhood, there did not appear a fair prospect of supporting a large family. In consequence, he and his wife determined to limit their offspring to three. They have accordingly used it for seven or eight years; have had no more children; and have been rewarded for their prudence by finding their situation and prospects improving every year.

The next communication from which we shall copy is from a young man of excellent character, living in a neighboring state, and now one of the conductors of a popular periodical. After suggesting to us the propriety of re-publishing some English works now out of print, he proceeds as follows:

"Had I not been addressing you upon another subject, I should not have ventured to obtrude on you my small meed of approbation; but I cannot let slip this opportunity of endeavoring to express how much I feel indebted to you for its publication.

"To know how I am so indebted, it is necessary you should also know something of my situation in life; and when it is described, it is perhaps a description of the situation of two-thirds of the journeymen mechanics of this country.

"I have been married nearly three years, and am the father of two children. Having nothing to depend upon but my own industry, you will readily acknowledge that I had reason to look forward with at least some degree of disquietude to the prospect of an increasing family and reduced wages: apparently the inevitable lot of the generality of working men.

"I had apparently nothing left but to let matters take their own course, when your valuable work made its appearance.

"I read it; and a new scene of existence seemed to open before me. I found myself, in this all-important matter, a free agent, and, in a degree, the arbiter of my own destiny

I could have said to you as Selim said to Hassan,—

'Thou'st hew'd a mountain's weight from off my heart.'

My visions of poverty and future distress vanished; the present seemed gilded with new charms, and the future appeared no longer to be dreaded. But you can better imagine, than I describe, the revolution of my feelings.

"I have since endeavored to circulate this book as widely as my limited opportunities permit, and shall continue to do so, believing it to be the most useful work that has made its appearance."

The next extract, from an inhabitant of Pennsylvania, we have selected chiefly as it furnishes a beautiful, and, alas! a rare, example, of that parental conscientiousness which scruples to impart existence where it cannot also impart the conditions necessary to render that existence happy. In this view, the control in question is indeed all-important. Were such virtue as this cultivated in mankind generally, how soon might the very seeds of disease die out among us, instead of bearing, as now, their poison-fruit fron generation to generation! and how far migh human beings, in succeeding ages, surpass their forefathers in strength, in health, and in beauty!

This view of the subject is to the physi

ologist, to the philosopher, to every friend of human improvement, a most interesting one. 'So long,' to use the words of an eloquent lecturer, 'as the tainted stream is unhesitatingly transmitted through the channel of nature, from parent to offspring, so long will the text be verified which "visits the sins of the fathers on the children, even to the third and fourth generation.'" And so long, we would add, will mankind—wise and successful whenever there is question of improving the animal races—be blind in perceiving, and listless in securing, that far nobler object, the physical, and thereby—in a measure—the mental and moral improvement of our own.

Here is the extract which led to these remarks:—

"I was born of poor parents, and early left an orphan. When of age, though my circumstances promised poorly for the support of a family, I desired to marry, knowing that a good wife would greatly add to my happiness. The preventive spoken of in your book presented itself to my mind, and for seven years that I have now been married, it has been used. I was successful in business, and acquired the means of maintaining a family; but still I have been unwilling, because my constitution is such a one as I think a parent ought not to transmit to his offspring. I prefer not to give birth to sentient beings, unless I can give them those advantages, physical as well as moral and intellectual, which are essential to human happiness."

From the letter of an aged French gentleman, who holds a public office in the western country, I translate the following; and would to heaven that every young man and woman in these United States could read it.

"I have read your work with much interest; and desire that it may have a wide circulation and that its recommendations may be adopted in practice. If you publish another edition, I could wish that you would add a piece of advice of the greatest importance, especially to young married persons. Many women are ignorant, that, in the gratification of the re-productive instinct, the exhaustion to the man is much greater than to the woman; a fact most important to be known, the ignorance of which has caused more than one husband to forfeit his health, nay, his life. Tissot tells us, that the loss by an ounce of semen is equal to that by forty ounces of blood;* and that, in the case of the healthiest man, nature does not demand connexion oftener than once a month.†

* "This, of course, must be rather a matter of conjecture and approximation, than of accurate calculation."

"† Any young man who will carefully note and compare his sensations, will become convinced, that temperance positively forbids such indulgence, at any rate, more than twice a week; and that he trifles with his con-

"How many young spouses, loving their husbands tenderly and disinterestedly, if they were but informed of these facts, would watch over and preserve their partners' healths, instead of exciting them to over-indulgence."—Another extract.

"A member of the Society of Friends, from the country, called at our office; he informed me that he had been married twenty years, had six children, and would probably have had twice as many, but for the preventive, which he found in every instance efficacious. By this means he made an interval of two or three years between the births of each of his children. Having at last a family of six, his wife earnestly desired to have no more; and on one occasion, when the preventive was neglected to be used, she shed tears at the prospect of again becoming pregnant. He said he knew, in his own neighborhood, several married women who were rendered miserable on account of their continued pregnancy, and would have given anything in the world to escape, but knew not how."

Our readers may implicitly depend on the

tution who neglects the prohibition. How immeasurably important that parents should communicate to their sons but especially to their daughters, facts like these! It is true that much depends upon habit, as some individuals can indulge even daily without apparently sustaining any physical injury; but such a frequency may not be compatible with the well-being of both parties. and should therefore not be encouraged."

accuracy of the facts we have stated. Though in the present state of public opinion we may not, for obvious reasons, give *names* in proof.

That most practical of philosophers, Franklin, interprets chastity to mean, *the regulated and strictly temperate satisfaction, without injury to others of those desires which are natural to all healthy adult beings.* In this sense, chastity is the first of virtues, and one most rarely practised, either by young men or by married persons, even when the latter most scrupulously conform to the letter of the law.

It is all important for the welfare of our race, that the re-productive instinct should never be selfishly indulged; never gratified at the expense of the well-being of our companions. A man who, in this matter, will not consult, with scrupulous deference, the slightest wishes of the other sex; a man who will ever put his desires in competition with theirs, and who will prize more highly the pleasure he receives than that he may be capable of bestowing—such a man appears to me, in the essentials of character, a brute The brutes commonly seek the satisfaction of their propensities with straight-forward selfishness, and never calculate whether their companions are gratified or teased by their importunities. Man cannot assimilate his nature more closely to theirs, than by imitating them in this.

Again. There is no instinct in regard to

which strict temperance is more essential. All our animal desires have hitherto occupied an undue share of human thoughts; but none more generally than this. The imaginations of the young and the passions of the adult are inflamed by mystery or excited by restraint, and a full half of all the thoughts and intrigues of the world has a direct reference to this single instinct. Even those, who like the Shakers, 'crucify the flesh,' are not the less occupied by it in their secret thoughts; as the Shaker writings themselves may afford proof. Neither human institutions nor human prejudices can destroy the instinct. Strange it is, that men should not be content rationally to control, and wisely to regulate it.

SEXUAL WEAKNESS.

This complaint, commonly called *fluor albus*, or *whites*, to which women are peculiarly subject, must form an important object of attention, since it is always attended with disagreeable symptoms; and, when aggravated, soon spoils the beauty of a fine face, weakens the digestive powers, produces a general bad habit, and occasions sterility.

Symptoms.

An irregular discharge from the passage leading to the womb, of a fluid, which, in different women, varies much in colour, being of a white, green, yellow, or brown hue. In the beginning it is, however, most usually white and pellucid, and, in progress of the complaint, acquires the various discolourations and different degrees of acrimony, whence proceed a slight smarting on making water. Besides the discharge, the patient is frequently afflicted with severe and constant pains in the back and loins, indigestion, paleness of the face, chilliness, and languor. In process of time, every symptom becomes highly aggravated, the feet and ankles swell, palpitations, and a difficulty of respiration are experienced, the menstrual discharge is rendered irregular, the urine is turbid, the mind is dejected, and either consumption or dropsy supervenes, and terminates a miserable existence.

In some languid habits, the fluor albus returns periodically, instead of the proper menstrual evacuation, until the patient's constitution is duly invigorated.

Causes.

It may be produced by any cause which either weakens or irritates the womb and its appendages. It may arise from general debility of the constitution, but it is especially caused by circumstances impairing the power of the womb itself, as, for instance, a severe labour, a miscarriage, or profuse menstruation.

In some instances it appears to depend on a full and irritable habit of body, and, in other cases, of local irritation, such as disorders of the womb, or of the urinary organs, or a collection in the gut, of the small thready worms called ascarides.

Upon the high authority of Dr. Hamilton, this disease is most frequently first brought on by some imprudence in respect to diet and clothing, or exposure to cold or fatigue, or neglect of the bowels about the time when menstruation begins.

Treatment.

In the treatment of this complaint regard must be had to the apparent cause, and to the state of the patient. The discharge is too often considered by the sex as the effects of general weakness in their habit, and, therefore, they are led to the indiscriminate use of heating medicines, as port wine, balsam copaibæ, &c., without paying attention to the habit of the body, or cause of the disease.

A milk diet, change of air, and the partial cold bath, as sponging the loins and thighs with cold water every morning, with attention to cleanliness and proper exercise, are often sufficient to arrest the disease, if early adopted.

In addition to this plan of treatment, if the patient be of a full habit, a disposition to fever from slight causes, attended with a sense of

necessary to have recourse to the lancet, cooling cathartics, and febrifuge medicines, and to inject, several times a day, flax-seed tea or milk and water, into the passage of the womb. In the great majority of cases, the complaint arises from general debility or laxity of the vessels of the parts, and in such cases the indications of cure are to increase the vital heat, promote the digestion, and restrain the preternatural discharge. In order to which, recourse must be had to such of the tonic medicines as will be found to agree best with the patient. Of these, the bark and elixir vitriol, the tonic powders or pills, the rust or tincture of steel, and lime-water have usually been employed, and often with good effects. In some instances, however, I have known these medicines to fail, when the nitric acid, diluted, in doses of a wine-glassful, three or four times a-day, wonderfully succeeded.

Previously to the exhibition of tonic medicines, it is advisable to give a dose of ipecacuanha or antimonial wine. Gentle emetics are supposed to be of singular utility in this complaint, not only by cleansing the stomach and bowels, and making a revulsion of the humors from the inferior part of the body, but likewise by their exciting all the powers of the constitution to a more vigourous action.

The bowels must be kept in a regular state by conjoining a few grains of rhubarb with some of the tonic medicines, or by taking occasionally, at bed-time, one of the aloetic, or aperient or diaphoretic pills; or, in the morning, a tea-spoonful of Epsom salts dissolved in a tumbler of water.

If there be a fulness of the stomach after eating, the tincture of rhubarb in small doses will excite digestion. In obstinate cases, it is often expedient to produce a change in the system, by giving a grain or two of calomel, r one of the mercurial pills at bed-time, until the gums become slightly affected, and then the cure may be completed by strengthening medicines, together with the shower bath.

Besides tonics, stimulating medicines, such

as commonly determine to the urinary passages, have very frequently been employed with great benefit. Of these, rosin in doses of ten grains in the yolk of an egg, or a spoonful of molasses, or balsam copaibæ in doses of a tea-spoonful, or tincture of cantharides in doses of twenty or thirty drops in some mucilaginous drink, and taken three or four times a day, will be found most salutary.

These means strike at the cause of the complaint; but if it do not remove the effect very soon, we are not to trust to them alone. For once a morbid secretion being excited, it is very apt to continue, although the exciting cause cease to operate.

On this account, we ought, without delay, to have recourse to astringent injections, such as a strong decoction of red oak bark, with the addition of a little alum or a solution of alum in water. Half an ounce of the former to be dissolved in a bottle of water: which should be thrown into the vagina by means of a female syringe, two or three times a day. The celebrated Dr. Burns says, after many trials, he satisfied himself, that although assistance may be derived from internal medicines and the cold bath, yet the chief dependence is to be placed on astringent applications to the seat of the discharge; and these, where there is no fulness of the general system, nor any affection of the womb itself, are perfectly safe, and seldom fail in producing a cure.

It will be prudent, when this disease occurs as an early symptom of pregnancy, not to check the discharge suddenly, lest miscar-rlage be the consequence: but it may be moderated by injections of water, with the addition of a little vinegar, or an infusion of green tea. Neither should the discharge be suddenly suppressed when it has been of long standing, and acquired a considerable degree of acrimony, with an offensive smell. For if it be unseasonably checked, the belly swells, and a train of the most disagreeable symptoms occurs. In such cases, soap-suds, or an infusion of chamomile flowers or hops, should be frequently thrown up the vagina; and, as soon as the blood is freed of its impurities, by suitable medicines, and has recovered, in some measure, its soft and balmy quality of which it has been deprived, the astringent injections may be employed with perfect safety.

The application of a blister to the sacrum, has, in some obstinate cases, been attended with advantage.

When the fluor albus proceeds from worms, purgatives and bitter clysters are the proper remedies.

Pain in the back and loins is often mitigated by the application of a large adhesive or strengthening plaster, and by avoiding a standing posture of long continuance, much walking, dancing, or any other violent exertion.

Women should carefully avoid all the remote causes of the disease: they should pay diligent attention to cleanliness, by washing the parts frequently with cold water; and when there are excoriations, milk and water, or lead-water, may be employed as a wash

Regimen.

The diet should be light, cordial, and nourishing, consisting of isinglass dissolved in milk by boiling it, jellies, custards, rice, milk, soft-boiled eggs, gelatinous broths, and light meats, together with a prudent use of genuine wine, particularly claret or port.

Women, affected with this disease, should by no means indulge in the use of tea and other warm slops of a relaxing nature; but should lie on a mattress in preference to a feather bed; and they should rise early, and take such daily exercise as their strength will admit, particularly on horseback. When there is much languor, with chilliness, friction with the flesh-brush, and wearing flannel next the skin, must not be omitted.

FALLING DOWN OF THE WOMB.

This is a much more common complaint than the former, and takes place in women of every age, and every rank. As its name implies, it consists of change in the situation of the womb, by which that organ lies much lower than it ought to do. In some cases it absolutely protrudes entirely without the parts. The slightest degrees are styled bearing down; and the more violent ones descent or falling down of the womb.

In general, the first symptom of this complaint is an uneasy sensation in the lower part of the back while standing or walking, with now and then a kind of pressure and bearing down.

If these feelings be disregarded, the complaint increases, and the patient becomes incapable of making water without first lying down, or pushing up a swelling which seems to stop the discharge of urine; and if the disease continues to increase, the womb is actually forced out of the parts, and takes on the form of a bulky substance hanging down between the thighs. This extreme degree of the complaint can seldom happen, excepting in women who have had a great many children, but the less degrees of it occur occasionally in very young unmarried women.

The causes of descent of the womb ought to be known to every woman, as many of them may be avoided. Every disease which induces weakness of the habit in general, or of the passage leading to the womb, in particular, must lay the foundation for the complaint. Frequent miscarriages, improper treatment duiing labour, too early or violent exercise after delivery, are in married women, the most frequent circumstances by which falling down of the womb is produced. In the unmarried, it is apt to take place in consequence of violent exercise, as in dancing, riding, &c., while out of order, a fact that ought to be impressed on the mind of every young woman.

In the treatment of this complaint, the means must be adapted to the degree of its violence. When the descent is inconsiderable, and the case is of recent date, the daily use of the cold bath, invigorating diet, very moderate exercise, and the injection of any mild astringent liquor into the passage, even ing and morning, will probably prove successful. But should the disease be in a great degree or of long standing, a course of tonics, with the frequent use of astringent injections, as a strong solution of alum in water, or decoction of red oak bark, must be added to the above means.

Dr. Leak advises, that after the parts are reduced, the intention of contracting the relaxed vagina so as to prevent its future descent, may be effected by the frequent use of the following astringent injection. Take of alum, and while vitriol, each, one drachm, boiling water, one pound, mix and filter through paper. Inject it into the vagina, milk warm, with a womb syringe. At the same time endeavour to strengthen the whole bodily system by nourishing diet, and tonic medicines.

When the complaint resists such remedies, or when, from its degree, it may appear unnecessary to employ them, the only relief which can be afforded, unless the womb become pregnant, is to be obtained by wearing an instrument called a pessary. It is made of wood or ivory, and if properly adapted to the passage, and of a proper construction, it can be worn without much inconvenience, and it never occasions pain. Certain attentions are however necessary, whenever such an instrument is used. Thus, the pessary should never be allowed to remain in the passage above a few days at a time, otherwise it becomes the source of great irritation. It should, therefore, be occasionally withdrawn on going to bed, well cleaned and reintroduced in the morning, before the patient rises. In some instances, after a pessary of a certain size has been worn for several months, one of a smaller size becomes better adapted to the passages, and in other cases one of a larger size is required.

Sponges of such a size as, when expanded fill up the cavity of the vagina, are very good *pessaries*. They support the uterus, and, by putting a string through them, the end of which is to be left hanging out of the os externum, the woman can take them away and apply them herself very conveniently.

To answer this purpose, a fine sponge,

wrung out in alum water, may be dried in a compressed state, and cut into any convenient form, so as to be introduced as high as possible: this will act by its astringency, and by its pressure, in a gentle and uniform manner. During the use of this application, an astringent injection may be used twice a day, and the sponge tent should be made gradually smaller as the vagina contracts.

The application of the bandage round the whole belly, with a moderate degree of firmness, often gives great relief to the uneasy feelings. The T bandage has also been worn in this case with considerable advantage.

If a woman liable to falling down of the womb, become pregnant, there is no occasion for the pessary after the third month, and by proper treatment after delivery, the return of the complaint may be prevented.

MISCARRIAGE OR ABORTION.

We now come to the consideration of a subject, in respect to which there exists much misapprehension and ignorance, causing useless and unnecessary alarm and anxiety to those who may be so unfortunate as to be subject, at particular periods of gestation, to abortion or miscarriage.

The dangers of abortion or miscarriage are often magnified and exaggerated. It is dangerous if produced by a fall, a blow, a kick from a horse, or any other external bodily violence or injury, causing internal contusion, or rupture of some blood vessels; and, also, but not to the same extent, if produced by sudden fright, violent fits of passion, &c., or from general debility or disease of the uterus; but the danger arises more from the cause which produces the miscarriage. than from the miscarriage itself; as it is well known by those versed in obstetrics that, where it is deemed indispensable to effect a miscarriage, either because of the existence of a deformed pelvis, diseased uterus, or other causes, if skilfully effected, it is attended with no danger, especially in the earlier stages of pregnancy.*

Symptoms.

When miscarriage is about to take place, its first symptoms are generally occasional stinging pains at the bottom of the belly, extending across and around the loins and hips; a feeling of fatigue of the legs, pain in the forehead, burning sensation of the eyes. The breasts, which before were distended, become soft and flabby, hot and cold flashes, attended with thirst, fever, and shiverings. In a day or two after the appearance of these symptoms, a discharge from the womb takes place of yellow matter, tinctured with red. If not arrested at this stage, the pains across the loins become more severe and frequent, attended with a sense of dead weight, and bearing down about the womb, the water is discharged, and the expulsion of the contents of the womb takes place. The symptoms of miscarriage, however, vary with the causes which produce them, or the state of habit.

* The writer, under the circumstances just mentioned, in the course of his practice as Professor of the Diseases of Women, has been called upon to effect miscarriages, and in all cases, it has proved perfectly safe recovery following in about three days. When necessary to be attended to, the earlier the better, but in no case if properly effected, with ordinary care on the part o the patient, is it attended with any danger. A skilfu and practised obstetrician will impart no pain

age, or health of the patient; some recovering immediately and rapidly, and with but little inconvenience. Where miscarriage arises from a serious accident, such as violent falls, bruises, &c., the symptoms are somewhat aggravated, and more severe, and are often preceded and accompanied with violent and profuse floodings and discharges of coagula, in addition to the other symptoms; although moderate flowing is not an unfrequent symptom in miscarriages.

It is always accompanied with two circumstances, separation of the membranous bag, and expulsive efforts or contraction of the womb itself. The first is productive of discharge, the second of pains like those of labor. Sometimes the separation or detachment of part of the conception takes place before any pain is felt; on other occasions, the pain, or contraction of the womb, takes place first, and produces a separation. In the first of these cases, the symptoms of abortion take place suddenly, and are usually occasioned by fatigue, sudden exertion, or fright. In the second, the pains come on, and there are particular feelings, and changes, which indicate that a miscarriage is likely to take place; as, for instance, the cessation of the morning sickness, the subsidence of the breasts, &c.

Miscarriage is preceded by floodings, pains in the back, loins, and lower part of the abdomen evacuation of the water, shiverings, palpitation of the heart, nausea, anxiety, fainting, subsiding of the breasts and belly, pain in the inside of the thighs, opening and moisture of the womb.

Causes.

The principal causes of miscarriage are blows or falls; great exertion or fatigue; sudden frights and other violent emotions of the mind; a diet too sparing or too nutritious; the abuse of spirituous liquors; other diseases, particularly fevers and hæmorrhages; likewise excessive bleeding, profuse diarrhœa or colic, particularly from accumulated fæces; immoderate venery, &c.

Treatment.

When a woman is threatened with a miscarriage, there are two objects to attend to; the first is, to prevent it if we can; the second is to manage it so that as little blood as possible be lost; and both these are obtained by the same means. With this view, the patient should immediately, on the first alarm, undress and go to bed, lightly covered, with a firm determination not to rise till the process be either checked or completely over. There should be little fire in the room, though it be winter; and in summer, the windows must be opened. Cloths wet with cold water, should instantly be applied to the lower part of the belly, and back: the drink must be cold, and everything stimulating should carefully be avoided.

In robust habits, or when the symptoms have been brought on suddenly by some such cause as a fall or exertion, it is proper to bleed; and, in cases of sickness or great feebleness, to give a dose of laudanum; or, what is better, to administer the anodyne clysters.*

Opiates are useful in every case where we hope to prevent abortion, and must be repeated more often or seldom, according to the effect they produce. They are, however improper in those cases where miscarriages must decidedly take place. Their tendency to occasion costiveness, when employed, must be obviated by clysters, or some gentle laxative medicine, such as calcined magnesia,

* *Anodyne Clyster.*—A gill of new milk, or thin starch, or the same quantity of any of the mucilaginous substances composing Simple and Emollient Clysters, which consist of milk and water in equal parts; flax-seed tea; infusion of quince-seed; barley water; mucilage of gum Arabic, or slippery elm; thin starch. From half a pint to a pint of either of these should be administered a little more than milk warm, with the addition of one or two tea-spoonfuls of laudanum, for adults. In general, patient will bear three times the quantity of laudanum administered in this way, than would be a proper dose when taken into the stomach: so that, when to procure rest, twenty-five drops would be given in a draught, seventy-five may be administered in a clyster, and the sickness, and other ill consequences, which some persons complain of after laudanum has been taken into the stomach, seldom follow when administered by clyster.

Epsom salts, or a little castor oil. If there be a continued but trifling discharge, great advantage may be derived from injecting, three or four times a day, up the vagina, a solution of alum. Indeed, in all protracted cases, this is of much benefit. The solution ought to be thrown up pretty high, that it may reach the womb.

When these means produce not the desired effect, and along with the discharge of blood large clots come off attended with bearing down or pains in the back and loins, especially if the symptoms which precede abortion have appeared, there must be every probability that the threatening event cannot be avoided; then we must conduct the patient through the process.

In all cases during the last stage of pregnancy, where our endeavors to stop or repress the hemorrhage prove abortive, it will be advisable to deliver her as soon as possible.

When the whole conception come away at once, the pain and discharge usually go off; but, if only the fœtus come away, all the symptoms either continue and increase till the placenta come away, or, if they be for a time suspended, they are sure to return, except in early miscarriages of ten or twelve weeks pregnancy, when sometimes the fœtus is expelled separately, and the placenta comes immediately after, but the latter frequently remains several days. The most prudent mode in such cases is to leave it to nature, which sooner or later expels this foreign body.

After the process is over, if the discharge be profuse, and do not stop on the application of cold water to the lower part of the belly, it will be proper to plug up the vagina, and this is best done by taking a piece of soft sponge, dipping it in sweet oil, and then wringing it gently. This is to be introduced with the finger, portion after portion, until the lower part of the vagina be well filled. The remainder is then to be firmly pressed on the orifice, and held there some time for the effused blood to coagulate. In obstinate cases, previously to the introduction of the plug, we may insert a little pounded ice, or snow tied up in a rag, if to be procured,* but neither of these should be continued so long as to produce pain or much shivering. In addition to this mode of treatment, it will be advisable to have recourse to the astringent medicines, as advised under the head of *Immoderate Flow of Menses.*

Regimen.

Arrow-root, tapioca, sago, panada, or rice milk, constitute a proper regimen. If the process be protracted, and the strength much impaired, the diet may be more liberal. In

* If faintness occurs from the loss of blood by flooding, a little brandy, with two-thirds cold water, should be given in frequent and small quantities at a time. Nothing so speedily restores the strength in such cases.

every case, ripe fruit is safe and useful. The bowels are to be kept regular, and sleep, if necessary, is to be procured by an anodyne.

Prevention.

It requires great attention to prevent abortion in subsequent pregnancies, whenever it has happened.

In all such cases, it will be highly necessary to attend to the usual habitudes and constitution of the woman, and to remove that condition which is found to dispose to abortion.

A woman that is subject to miscarriage, and who is of a full plethoric habit, ought to take the tincture of foxglove, twice or thrice a day, for two or three weeks.

She should likewise keep her body perfectly open with gentle aperient medicines, use a spare diet, and avoid all agitations of the mind. The sleep should be abridged in quantity, and taken on a mattress, instead ot a feather bed. Regular and moderate exercise should be taken daily, being cautious, at the same time, not to carry it to the length ol exciting fatigue.

In women of a weak, lax habit, a nutritive and generous diet, moderate exercise, and tonic medicines, will be required. And, along with nourishing diet, a moderate use of wine should be allowed, if it do not heat the patient, or otherwise disagree. The cold bath is of signal service in every instance where it is not followed by chilliness.

Until gestation be far advanced, it would be advisable for the woman to sleep alone, and strictly avoid every cause which is ascertained to be capable of producing abortion.

Women more frequently miscarry in the second or third month than at any other time; but some have a certain period at which they usually go wrong, and do not vary a week from it. In such cases, the woman should confine herself to the house, avoid the least exercise, and frequently recline on the sofa or bed, till that period be past.

When a female has suffered several abortions, it becomes almost impossible to prevent a repetition at the same period of gestation in a subsequent pregnancy. Nothing, however, will be so successful in preventing a recurrence of a similar misfortune, as in allowing the uterine vessels to recover their tone; for which purpose tonics must be given Attend to particular symptoms as they occur; with proper diet and exercise. *Sea Bathing* and the *shower bath* are both excellent.*

* As in most cases the predisposition to miscarry arises from a very weakened or diseased state of the uterus, or general debility of the system, which is mostly caused by one period of pregnancy followed by miscarriage, too closely succeeding another with the same results, it is

When necessary to effect Miscarriage or Artificial Delivery.

During pregnancy, deformities of the pelvis become objects of solicitude to the accoucheur, when they are of such a character as to render delivery at full term impossible without the interference of cutting operations. At this period only can he guard against the deplorable consequences of these deformities.

Pelvic Deformities.

The accoucheur may be consulted by a mother anxious to know whether the pelvis of her daughter is such as to justify marriage. His opinion may also be desired by a female pregnant for the first time, in whose mind there may exist fears as to the formation of her pelvis. In this case, he will have to reply to the following questions:

Is delivery at full term compatible with the safety of the child? What influence will the deformity have on pregnancy? What precautions are necessary to guard against

obvious that the prevention of pregnancy by the use of M. Desomeaux's "*Preventive of Pregnancy,*" (treated of in the preceding pages,) for about two years or so, or until health and strength are restored, is the proper remedy; thereby enabling the system to correct the predisposition, by improving the tone and vigour of the uterus. The writer can vouch that by the use of this "Preventive," many women who had before constantly miscarried, at particular periods, entirely recovered, and gave birth to full grown and healthy children, after trying all other means without avail.

accident until the completion of gestation, and to facilitate delivery?

When the accoucheur states that delivery will not be possible without the interference of art, he will then be asked whether this interference will compromise the life of th mother or child; and whether this operation cannot be avoided by some process during pregnancy, either saving the life of mother and child, or sacrificing the child for the benefit of the mother?

In order to answer these questions satisfactorily, and to furnish himself with a rule of conduct in advance, it will be necessary for the accoucheur to know precisely the condition of the pelvis, and the dimensions of the diameters, &c.

However, it must not be supposed that this mensuration can be made with mathematical accuracy; our means will not enable us to obtain this precision; but even if we could, the object we have in view would not be completely accomplished, for, in order to arrive at a rigorous appreciation of the consequences of the deformity and the operations it might require, it would be necessary also to know the exact size of the fœtus, which is not possible.

Happily, in practice, an approximation as to the absolute condition of the pelvis will suffice, and it is easy to arrive at this result. With this view, the accoucheur should, in the first place, learn the previous history of the patient in infancy and youth, and afterward proceed to an external and internal examination.

When the accoucheur is called upon to pass an opinion as to the natural or unnatural onformation of a female, he should, says M. P. Dubois, inquire minutely into the antecedent condition of this woman during her infancy and youth. The history of early life will often, of itself, cause him to suspect the state of the pelvis. He should address the following questions to the parent:

What diseases was the infant affected with? At what age did they manifest themselves? At what age did the child walk? After walking, did it appear weak in the inferior extremities? Was the erect position possible? Was it easy? Were the articulations large?

If all these phenomena appeared in infancy, it is highly probable that the pelvis is deformed; and, moreover, it may be affirmed that the symptoms arose from rickets, a disease peculiar to infancy. It commences rarely before eighteen or twenty months, and very seldom after thirteen or fourteen years of age. If there should be curvatures of the spinal column and extremities, it will be almost certain that the pelvis is deformed; and if the curvature commenced in the inferior extremities, we may conclude that it is owing to rachitis, for this disease exerts its influence first on the tibias, then on the bones of the thighs, pelvis, and vertebral column. On the contrary, if the first ten years have been passed without disturbance of the general health, then curvatures must be attributed to malacosteon, especially if the curvature of the spine has preceded that of the lower limbs. Deformity of the spine may exist alone; then we may legitimately hope that the pelvis is not contracted. Experience, indeed, proves that the vertebral column may be considerably curved without the pelvis participating in the deformity, when the inferior extremities are straight; and that, in general, curvatures of the extremities alone accompany pelvic malformations.

Indeed, it is not on simple probabilities that the accoucheur is to interdict the marriage* of a young girl, or determine, during pregnancy, to perform an operation, with the view of protecting the mother against the dangers of delivery at full term.

Premature Artificial Delivery.

Thanks to the efforts of MM. Stoltz Dezeimeris, P. Dubois, and Velpeau, delivery brought on before the full term is an operation hereafter recognised in French midwifery. For a long time it proved useful to ur neighbors in England and Germany, while a foolish prejudice caused it to be re-

* Interdiction of marriage is not necessary, all that is required is that *pregnancy should be prevented;* this, thanks to M. Desomeaux's discovery can be attained bv the use of his "Preventive to Pregnancy."

jected by French practitioners, who did not hesitate even to have recourse to the Cæsarean section and symphyscotomy.

We have not within the walls of Paris one solitary example of a woman who had survived the Cæsarean section. She who lived the longest was one of those on whom I assisted M. P. Dubois to operate. She died on the seventeenth day of a tetanic affection, when everything promised a most successful result.—(*Bull. of the Acad. of Med.*, t. iii., p. 694; . v., p. 25.

Whent the contraction is such that a living fœtus cannot be brought forth, the accoucheur has then to choose between the Cæsarean section or miscarriage.

During pregnancy, abortion will present an extreme and last resource. And it would seem more humane to sacrifice, before the period of viability, an embryo whose existence is so uncertain, in order to protect the mother from the perilous chances of symphyscotomy and the Cæsarean section.

I must confess that, if such an alternative were presented to me, the diameter of the pelvis being only two inches, I should not hesitate to propose this means.

The abuse and criminal extension of such a resource is reprehensible, but not its proper and authorized employment. This operation should always be undertaken with great care, and all necessary precaution used to satisfy the public mind of its necessity.

16

LABOR, DELIVERY, ETC

After seven months of pregnancy the fœtus has all the conditions for breathing and exercising its digestion. It may then be separated from its mother, and change its mode of existence. Child-birth rarely, however, happens at this period: most frequently the fœtus remains two months longer in the uterus, and it does not pass out of this organ till after the revolution of nine months.

Examples are related of children being born after ten full months of gestation; but these cases are very doubtful, for it is extremely difficult to know the exact period of conception. The legislation in France, however, has fixed the principle, that child-birth may take place up to the two hundred and ninety-ninth day of pregnancy.

Nothing is more curious than the mechanism by which the fœtus is expelled; everything happens with wonderful precision; all seems to have been foreseen, and calculated to favor its passage through the pelvis and the genital parts.

The physical causes that determine the exit of the fœtus are the contraction of the uterus and that of the abdominal muscles;

by their force the liquor amnii flows out, the head of the fœtus is engaged in the pelvis, it goes through it, and soon passes out by the valve, the folds of which disappear; these different phenomena take place in succession and continue a certain time; they are accompanied with pains more or less severe; with swelling and softening of the soft parts of the pelvis and external genital parts, and with an abundant mucous secretion in the cavity of the vagina. All these circumstances, each in its own way, favor the passage of the fœtus. To facilitate the study of this action, it may be divided into several periods.

The first period of child-birth.—It is constituted by the precursory signs. Two or three days before child-birth a flow of mucus takes place from the vagina, the external genital parts swell and become softer; it is the same with the ligaments that unite the bones of the pelvis; the mouth of the womb flattens, its opening is enlarged, its edges become thinner; slight pains, known under the name of *flying pains*, are felt in the loins and abdomen.

Second period.—Pains of a peculiar kind come on; they begin in the lumbar region, and seem to be propagated towards the womb or the *rectum;* and are renewed only after intervals of a quarter or half an hour each. Each of them is accompanied with an evident contraction of the body of the uterus, with tension of its neck and dilatation of the opening; the finger directed into the vagina discovers that the envelopes of the fœtus are pushed outward, and that there is a considerable tumor, which is called *the waters* the pains very soon become stronger, and the contraction of the uterus more powerful; the membranes break, and a part of the liquid escapes; the uterus contracts on itself, and is applied to the surface of the fœtus.

Third period.—The pains and contractions of the uterus increase considerably; they are instinctively accompanied by the contraction of the abdominal muscles. The woman who is aware of their effect is inclined to favour them, by making all the muscular efforts of which she is capable: her pulse then becomes stronger and more frequent; her face is animated, her eyes shine, her whole body is in extreme agitation, and perspiration flows in abundance. The head descends into the lower strait of the pelvis.

Fourth period.—After some moments of repose the pains and expulsive contractions resume all their activity; the head presents itself at the vulva, makes an effort to pass, and succeeds when there happens to be a contraction sufficiently strong to produce this effect. The head being once disengaged, the remaining parts of the body easily follow, on account of their smaller volume

The section of the umbilical cord is then made, and a ligature is put around it at a short distance from the umbilicus or navel.

Fifth period.—If the midwife has not proceeded immediately to the extraction of the placenta after the birth of the child, slight pains are felt in a short time, the uterus contracts freely, but with force enough to throw off the placenta and the membranes of the ovum; this expulsion bears the name of *delivery*. During the twelve or fifteen days that follow child-birth the uterus contracts by degrees upon itself, the woman suffers abundant perspirations, her breasts are extended by the milk that they secrete; a flow of matter, which takes place from the vagina, called *lochia*, first sanguiferous, then whitish, indicates that the organs of the woman resume, by degrees, the disposition they had before conception.

MANAGEMENT OF LABOR.

Women in general are ignorant of parturition or delivery. Almost all of them are under the impression that labor is completed more by art than nature; hence the most noted accoucheurs are employed to attend during this interesting period; and professional men, in general, have no wish to undeceive them on this subject, as their interest is too much concerned. It is often astonishing to see the credulity and ignorance manifested on these occasions. Thanks and blessings have been poured forth, under the idea that he had saved their lives in labor, when the accoucheur had merely looked on nd admired the perfectly adequate powers of nature, and superintended the efforts of her work; and it is nature that accomplishes all, while the accoucheur gets the credit of it. There is not one case in a thousand in which he can do more than remain a silent spectator, except to calm the fears of the ignorant and timid attendants. The mischief and injury that are done by the untimely interference of art are incalculable.

In pregnancy women are bled till they have not strength enough to accomplish delivery; and, when it takes place, the forceps or other instruments are used, which often prove fatal to the mother or child, or both.

There are various particulars to be avoided, and several things to be done, in the management of women during labor. We have room here to state only a few, and shall begin by pointing out the course to be pursued in

Natural Labor.

When called to a woman supposed to be in labor, ascertain if her pains are *true* or *false*, which may be easily known by a little inquiry. If the female complains of flying or unsettled pains about the system, occurring mostly toward evening or during the night, and being slight or irregular, it may be taken for granted that they are spurious or false. If these symptoms prove troublesome, an infusion or tea of *hops* may be taken; or, if this is not sufficient to relieve them, or procure sleep, an anodyne may be taken; and it may be necessary also to give laxative medicines or an injection, with a little laudanum.

True pains may be known by the pain being more concentrated in the lower part of the belly, through the loins and hips.

The pains now increase in regularity and force, returning every ten or fifteen minutes, and leaving the woman comparatively easy in the intervals.

When the pains become regular and severe, there is a discharge of slimy matter, tinged with blood, known by the name of *shows*. At this period of labor it will be proper for the person who attends the labor to examine, in order to ascertain what part of the child presents, which may be done by requesting the female to sit in the chair or on the side of the bed, and to extend the legs when the longest finger, dipped in sweet oil, may be passed up the vagina to the part which presents, and the sense communicated will determine the nature of the presentation. In nineteen cases out of twenty, or in almost every case, the head will be felt. Frequent examinations should be avoided.

Dr. Bard, speaking of examinations, remarks: "What terms shall I use to condemn, as it deserves, the abominable practice of boring, scooping, and stretching the soft parts of the mother, under the preposterous idea of making room for the child to pass. It is impossible to censure this dangerous practice too severely; it is always wrong; nor can there be any one period in labor, the most easy and natural, the most tedious and difficult, the most regular or preternatural in which it can be of the least use; in which it will not unavoidably do great mischief: it will render an easy labor painful; one which would be short, tedious; and one which, if left to nature, would terminate happily, highly dangerous."

"All that is proper to be done in a case of natural labor, from its commencement to its termination," says Dr. McNair, "will suggest itself to any person of common understanding; and I have long labored under the conviction, that the office of attending women in their confinement should be intrusted to prudent females. There is not, according to my experience, and the reports of the most eminent surgeons, more than one case in three thousand that requires the least assistance. I am aware, however, that there are crafty physicians who attempt, and often succeed, in causing the distressed and alarmed female to believe that it would be altogether impossible for her to get over her troubles without their assistance; and, for the purpose of making it appear that their services are absolutely necessary, they will be continually interfering, sometimes with their instruments when there is not the least occasion for it. There is no doubt in my mind but that one-half of the women attended by these men are delivered before their proper period; and this is the reason why we see so many deformed children, and meet with so many females who have incurable complaints."

It is a very common circumstance for an inexperienced (or he may be an experienced, but ignorant) practitioner to attempt a rupture of the membranes, and in doing so, rupture the bladder, which would render the woman miserable during life. We are acquainted with twenty-five or thirty females who have met with this sad misfortune, and many of them have been attended by those who are termed our most successful, or old experienced physicians.

Dr. Rush, speaking of child-bearing among the Indians, says, "that nature is their only *midwife*; their labors are short and accompanied with little pain; each woman is delivered in a private cabin, without so much as one of her own sex to attend her: after washing herself in cold water, she returns in a few days to her usual employment; so that she knows nothing of those accidents which proceed from the carelessness or ill management of *midwives* or doctors, or the weakness which arises from a month's confinement in a warm room."

Dr. Whitney remarks; "I have had many cases where I found the attendants alarmed, and some in tears, from supposing that they should have had help sooner, fearing the worst consequence from delay; but, admitting that the 'doctor knew best,' they would wait calmly for hours, when in nature's time all ended well. I pledge myself as a physician, that all honest doctors will tell you that *labor* is the work of *nature*, and she generally does it *best* when left to herself."*

"Among the Araucanian Indians," says Stevenson in his Twenty Years' Residence in South America, "a mother, immediately on her delivery, takes her child, and going down to the nearest stream, washes herself and it, and returns to the usual labor of her station."

"The wonderful facility with which the Indian women bring forth their children," say Lewis and Clark in their well known journal, "seems rather some benevolent gift of nature, in exempting them from pains which their savage state would render doubly grievous, than any result of habit One of the women who had been leading two of our pack horses, halted at a rivulet

*This is true when it is a right presentation (the head) or when the duration and severity of labor may not induce convulsions

about a mile behind, and sent on the two horses by a female friend. On enquiring of one of the Indian men the cause of her detention, he answered, with great appearance of unconcern, that she had just stopped to lie in, and would soon overtake us. In fact we were astonished to see her in about an hour's time come on with her new-born infant, and pass us on her way to the camp, apparently in perfect health."

Washington Irving, in his work entitled Astoria, relates a similar incident in the following language: "The squaw of Pierre Dorion (who, with her husband, was attached to a party travelling over the Rocky Mountains in winter-time, the ground being covered with several feet of snow) was suddenly taken in labor, and enriched her husband with another child. As the fortitude and good conduct of the woman had gained for her the good will of the party, her situation caused concern and perplexity. Pierre, however, treated the matter as an occurrence that could soon be arranged, and need cause no delay. He remained by his wife in the camp, with his other children and his horse, and promised soon to rejoin the main body on their march. In the course of the following morning the Dorion family made its appearance. Pierre came trudging in advance, followed by his valued, though skeleton steed, on which was mounted his squaw with the new-born infant in her arms, and her boy of two years old wrapped in a blanket, and slung on her side. The mother looked as unconcerned as if nothing had happened to her; so easy is nature in her operations in the wilderness, when free from the enfeebling efinements of luxury and the tampering appliances of art."

When it has been ascertained that the labor is natural, or that there are no impediments or obstacles, there will be very little more to do than superintend the process. It will be necessary to give instructions to the attendants to make suitable preparation, or have everything required in readiness.

The woman may be delivered upon a bed or a cot, as is most convenient; if a bed be used, all but the mattress should be turned back toward the head, and it should be so prepared that the moisture from the uterus and other discharges may not add to the discomfort of the woman. A dressed skin, oilcloth, or folded blanket may be placed on that part of the mattress on which the body of the woman is to rest; a coarse blanket folded within a sheet, ought to be laid immediately beneath the patient, to absorb the moisture, which must be removed after delivery; the rest of the bed-clothes are to be put on in the ordinary way. The woman when she is no longer able to remain up may lie down, with her head elevated in any position which is most desirable; and in nearly every case that I have ever attended the back has been preferred, although most all writers recommend that the woman be placed upon her side: the latter practice is unnatural and wrong, for obvious reasons; it retards the labor pains, and prevents the midwife from superintending the progress of the labor; the pillow that is directed to be placed between the knees, to keep them widely separated, soon gets displaced by the motion or change of the female; and the legs, instead of being kept apart, again come in contact, and thus the passage of the child is obstructed: but when the female is placed upon her back this difficulty is obviated, a free passage is permitted, the pains are more effectual, the spine is better supported, and better access can be had to the parts during labor and after the delivery of the child; in short, there is a decided advantage in this position in every respect.

The dress of women in labor should be light and simple, both to keep themselves from being overheated, and to prevent anything from being in the way of what assistance is necessary. In addition to the means recommended, I direct a sheet to be placed around the waist of the woman, to prevent the blood excrements or waters from coming in contact with the linen or clothes, and, as much as possible, the bed; her linen may be tucked or pushed up so far that there will be no necessity of a removal after delivery.

Every thing being thus adjusted, very lit

tle more will be necessary but to wait patiently the efforts and operations of nature. There should be but few attendants in the room, and these are not to whisper to each other, or to express any fears or doubts.

A humane midwife will use every ingenious effort in her power to quiet the useless fears, and support and comfort the patient. A crowd of frightened, hysterical women, assailing the ears of the woman with tales of woe and sad disasters that have happened should be admonished. Half a dozen midwives, each making pretensions to great skill, ambition, and competition for obstetric fame, assembled around a feeble woman when labor is of a lingering character, is always an unfortunate circumstance, and it would be much better if nearly every one were afar off.

When the pains become very severe, quickly succeeding each other, the midwife, or the person who officiciates, may sit by the side of the woman, and, upon every severe pain, may keep her hand upon the parts, even though no manner of assistance can be afforded, and occasionally, when the head of the child presses hard, it may be gently touched or pressed with the longest finger, in order to ascertain the parts that prevent the progress of labor, as well as to be able to give from time to time suitable encouragement: not only so; in the last stage of labor the hand may be kept near the parts, to know the moment when the head of the child presents, as some little assistance at this time is called for; but not by supporting the perinæum, as some advise, but,

First. To remove any obstruction which often arises from the clothes.

Second. To support the child in its passage, and in the interval of pains; and to keep the head from pitching downward, and thus obstructing the labor.

Third. To detach the umbilical cord or navel-string from the neck when it encircles it, as is often the case, and which endangers the life of the child.

Fourth. To deliver the woman in case of hemorrhage or great flooding; but at the same time there must be no further interference of art; little or nothing can be done toward facilitating the delivery of the child except when a large bag or collection of water presents and opposes, when it may be ruptured with the longest finger, which often affords much aid, although such is the ignorance and credulity of some women, that they suppose almost everything to be accomplished by art. Physicians or midwives who watch only the process of labor, and do little or nothing, are pronounced inhuman and cruel, and perhaps ignorant, because they are honest in not interfering with the simple and beautiful process of labor, or in other words, for relying upon the great resources of nature: but such is the fashion and credulity of mankind, or rather womankind, that physicians are obliged to take the advantage of such ignorance and credulity, and regulate their proceedings accordingly. We have often been obliged to stand for hours over a woman, under pretence of aiding delivery, when, in *reality*, we did nothing at all. The abor would have progressed just as well had we been out of the room; but this deception we have been obliged to practise, in order to satisfy ignorant, gossiping, or crying attendants. When the woman is disposed to make much noise, she should be directed to hold her breath during the pains, and aid or assist them by pressing downward as much as possible. The feet may press against the bed-post, and the woman take hold of a handkerchief and pull when a pain occurs; or she may grasp the hand of an assistant for that purpose. Sometimes, from various causes, labor is very much retarded, from rigidity of the parts, the situation of the child, debility, &c.; when this occurs, and labor is tedious and protracted, our reliance must still be upon the powers of nature. We may, however, aid her efforts, by warm fomentations of *bitter herbs*, often applied to the lower part of the belly, which will prove relaxing, and will facilitate the labor; warm diluent drinks may also be given, such as *tansy*, *pennyroyal*, *&c.*

If the labor still continues stationary, we have nothing to fear, provided there is a right presentation; but should the pains become feeble or lessened from flooding, debility, or any cause, or should they prove unavailable, after a reasonable length of time, a drachm of *spurred rye* or *ergot* may be put into a tea-cup, and a gill of boiling water poured upon it, and, when cool, a table-spoonful given every fifteen minutes. This will increase the pains, and speedily accomplish a delivery; but it should be very seldom, or never, used, except when there is a right presentation, and under the most urgent circumstances.

It is prudent, by judicious precaution and care, to remove obstructions, prevent accidents by holding or supporting the child in a proper position, and giving such aid as reason and judgment will dictate. Receiving the child, preventing its fall, securing the navel cord, assisting in the removal and disposal of the after-birth, are objects which are to be accomplished, and all in the most calm and simple manner; no hurry or excitement is necessary, but, on the contrary, they embarrass. Yet how common is it that females in general, married and unmarried, are so uninformed and ignorant, that, instead of attending to those duties, if necessary, or in cases of emergency, they are thrown into the greatest consternation, and perhaps run out of the room and let the child suffocate by the bed-clothes, or by the navel cord twisted about the neck, and die merely for the want of a little common sense and knowledge, which might be acquired in an hour. Is it not highly disgraceful, if not criminal, that farmers can, and do, attend to those duties toward their stock, and yet remain entirely ignorant of them toward their nearest relations? Young women and men are taught music, dancing, drawing, needle-work, and many ornamental branches considered so essential to a polite education; yet they are suffered to remain entirely ignorant on a subject of so much vital importance. Is there any hope or prospect of enlightening this generation, or must it be delayed till the next, and have them look back with amazement at our ignorance? We hope there is something yet redeeming in a large proportion of the community; that the people will yet awake to their own interests.

When the head is delivered, all that is necessary to do is, to support it, and wait for the pains to expel the child; except it seems livid and in danger of injury, or when the cord is twisted around the neck, when assistance must be rendered, to accomplish the delivery. The face of the child must now be turned upward, and the cord freed from the neck or body; the person who assists will pass a narrow piece of tape around the cord or navel-string, about an inch from the body, and tie as tight as it can be drawn, otherwise hemorrhage or bleeding will take place; and another must be tied at a little distance from it, above, and be separated between them with a pair of scissors. The child is then to be given to the nurse, to be washed, dried and dressed. The woman must now be covered, and directed to lie quiet.

The After-birth.—The after-birth or placenta must be detached or removed, if nature does not accomplish it in a short time. Generally, after about twenty or thirty minutes, a pain is felt, which may be sufficient to expel it; if it should not, and should there be no pain, gentle manual attempts may be made to remove it.

The head and breast may be elevated, and the cord taken hold of by the left hand: the two first fingers may be carefully introduced into the vagina, and the anterior or forepart of the placenta or after-birth held in this situation for some minutes, in order to excite a contraction of the uterus. The woman may now be directed to hold her breath and press down, which forces it forward; and at the same time a little extension may be made upon the cord with the left hand, while extension is made upon the after-birth with the right; this will almost invariably extract it in a few minutes. If from any cause it should not, no farther attempts must be made for the present, but left for a few hours. when, if the natural contractions of the uterus do not remove it, it must be done in the manner recommended, with this difference, that a little more force be used. In the interval.

howevei, everything wet must be taken away.

Subsequent Treatment.—After the labour has been thus completed, if the woman is not too weak, assistants may raise her up, and seat her upon the side of the bed or cot, while another removes all the wet clothing from the patient and her bed, and with a little warm spirits washes off the blood, water, &c., that remain on her person. This is particularly necessary, as the omission of it may give rise to puerperal fever. We know not that others have practised this method; but we have found it conducive to the comfort as well as the health of the patient. Some practitioners will not suffer the woman to be removed from the situation in which she has been delivered under twelve or twenty-four hours, for fear of hemorrhage or flooding; but this is a great and dangerous error. It is impossible to tell what mischief may arise in consequence of suffering her to remain drenched in water and blood for this length of time.

After these precautions have been observed, and the bed properly prepared, on which has been placed folded blankets, skin, or oil-cloth, covered with a warm sheet, she may be laid down, and a diaper or suitable piece of muslin laid to the parts to absorb the lochial discharges. A bandage may be also placed around the abdomen or belly, and made moderately tight, but not so as to render her uncomfortable. A large tub, previously well dried, may be placed by the side of the bed, and the woman directed to place her feet in it, and, when she is lifted up, everything that is around her wet to be passed into it. It prevents the necessity of afterward washing the floor and carpet. which might prove injurious by causing a check to perspiration.

Preternatural labor, or cross-births, are those in which some other part than the head presents. We cannot in general assign any reason for such occurrences, nor can the woman, by any sensation of her own, be assured that the presentation is unusual. Apprehensions of this kind should not be indulged in. If the feet or breech present, the delivery is to be accomplished by properly accommodating the position of the child to the capacity of the pelvis, but no force should be employed; and though there is always some risk to the life of the infant, yet there is none to the mother. If the arm, shoulder, or sides of the child present, the delivery is not impossible, but difficult, until the infant be turned and the feet brought down into the passage. This is an operation which may be done with comparative ease and safety, if the wrong position of the infant be discovered before the waters are discharged; but other wise both mother and child are in considerable danger, though there is often a spontaneous evolution and delivery is effected. The womb closely contracting round the body of the infant when the water is drained away and being soft and spongy in its texture, it is liable to be torn if much force be employed, and then either the child may escape into the cavity of the belly, or, if it be extracted by the feet, blood may be effused from the womb into that cavity, and such injury be done as to prove fatal. Women too frequently add to the danger of the operation of turning, by their restlessness and impatience ; they should remember how much is at stake, and exert all their fortitude, so as not to embarrass the practitioner.

The labor having been thus accomplished, it will be necessary to guard against any subsequent symptoms which may occur or take place.

In *tedious* and very *difficult* labors, and where common physicians use the lancet, the hot bath will be found of extraordinary benefit in facilitating labor, by its relaxing the system without debility; altogether better than bleeding. First apply spirits, water, and salt to the head ; then let the woman continue in the bath about fifteen minutes.

Still-born Infants.—This occurs from difficult labors, or the cord encircling the neck ; or a membrane may cover the head or body. When anything of the kind occurs, the membrane should be immediately removed. If no signs of life appear, the infant may be put into the warm bath, and the mouth and body wiped dry. A little cold water may be dashed into the face, the lungs inflated by some person, and a slight motion made upon the chest in imitation of breathing. The navel-string may be permitted to bleed a little.

TREATMENT AFTER DELIVERY.

After-pains.—Soon after delivery these usually come on, and with some women prove remarkably severe. The quicker the labor has been, the slighter will they prove in general. Women with their first child are seldom much troubled with after-pains; but as the uterus is thought to contract less readily after each future labor, so they are more liable to suffer from them in any succeeding delivery than in the first.

When after-pains prove so troublesome as to deprive the patient of her rest, it will be necessary to have recourse to *fomentations* or *anodynes;* red pepper and spirits, simmered together a few minutes, and flannels dipped in it and applied to the belly, will generally relieve them; if it fails, apply a fomentation of *bitter herbs*, and give two teaspoonfuls of the tincture of *hops* in milk or tea. If these fail, which I never knew, give half a teaspoonful of *capsicum* in milk. These remedies are to be assisted by keeping up a sufficient pressure on the belly at the ame time by means of a broad bandage

---

NURSING

A CHILD must not be put to the breast, it the mother's health is very poor, or if she has any venereal, scrofulous, consumptive taint, or herpetic disease, St. Anthony's fire, &c. We have conversed with females who are subject to the last complaint, and who have communicated it to their children, which destroyed them all. The poison is transmitted from the mother to the child. In any of these cases, the infant must be reared on the nursing bottle. It is best to use cream instead of milk; the child thrives well upon it, less quantity answers, and it does not curdle, like milk, upon the stomach.

Atrophy from Suckling.—Some women of a delicate constitution cannot suckle long without an evident appearance of declining health; and, if persisted in, it might terminate in a general wasting of the body and loss of strength, or some morbid affection of the lungs. When, therefore, a woman finds her health declining, and that she gets weaker every day with loss of appetite and languor, she ought immediately to leave off suckling; she should use a generous diet, with a moderate quantity of wine bitters daily, and, if convenient, change the air, particularly if an inhabitant of a large and populous city or town. If the change is not found sufficiently efficacious of itself, when conjoined with a restorative diet, a course of *tonics* should be given. Gentle exercise on horseback or in a carriage will greatly assist the effect of these remedies.

INFLAMMATION OF THE BREASTS.

THIS disease is easily known by the pain, hardness, and swelling which accompany it. In some cases the whole breast appears to be affected; in others, only on one side and, in some, the effect is small and superficial.

When the breast inflames, it is evident that the retention of the milk must, for a time at least, increase the pain.

The first object then should be to have the breasts drawn, either by the child or some other means; but, should the milk not come away readily, and the pain be increased thereby, farther attempts must not be made; otherwise both the disease and sufferings of the woman may be aggravated. A cooling diet and an open state of the bowels are necessary while the swelling continues. And it is better for the patient to remain in bed, as the weight of the breast, while in the erect posture, often increases the inflammation. The breast should be gently rubbed with a small quantity of sweet oil or unsalted butter, and poultices of crumb of bread and lead water applied. If the pain and hardness do not very soon go off by this application, warm emollient poultices, as milk and bread, with a little oil, or united with the leaves of the thorn apple, must be had recourse to. These poultices will not promote suppuration unless the inflammation has proceeded so far, that the process has already begun, and in this case the sooner it is produced the better.

If the abscess do not point and break soon, no good can be gained by delay: an opening should therefore be made, so as to evacuate the matter freely. This not only gives immediate relief, but prevents a farther extension of the mischief. The milk and bread or flax-seed poultices must be continued for a few days, in order to remove the hardness, and then the part must be dressed, as in ordinary cases.

Indurations remaining after an abscess, may be frequently remedied by the application of a mercurial plaster, or cloths wet with the camphorated spirit, or rubbing the part, night and morning, with mercurial ointment, united with a little camphor.

Sometimes after the abscess heals, and the breast seems to be cured, it swells a little, especially towards night. This is from weakness, and is cured by strengthening the constitution.

Many women suffer more from this complaint than from all the various stages of pregnancy, labor, and delivery combined, and with whom broken breasts are an invariable attendant of confinement; they overlook all the other sufferings they have to undergo, and fix their dread and apprehension upon this. It is, therefore, all-important *that inflammation of the breasts should not be permitted to take place*, by proper precautionary measures, *and this can, in all cases, be accomplished*, by the mode of treatment pointed out in this work, which, as yet, has not been mentioned in any other, but of its invariable success there is not a shadow of doubt, as it has been tested under circumstances the most unfavorable, in cases where every confinement was attended with broken breasts, till this mode of treatment was had recourse to, and the patients, to their great surprise and joy, for the first time entirely escaped their uniform affliction. It is hoped the medical faculty will avail themselves of this invaluable mode of treatment, that hereafter inflammation of the breasts may be unknown, since prevention is so easy and practicable.

To prevent Inflamed or Broken Breasts.

This most desirable and important object is accomplished by covering the entire breasts with diacylon plaster (which can be obtained of every druggist, the machine-spread is preferable) rather tightly or closely put on, merely making a round hole (about the circumference of a dollar) for the nipple, sufficiently large not to interfere with the suckling of the infant, should it be put to the breast; and if not, it is not only unnecessary to draw the milk, but it would be advisable to refrain from it, even if a little pain or distension should supervene, as the milk is sure to find an outlet in the nipple. The plaster must be cut round and embrace and cover the entire of each breast, and should be put on within eight or ten hours after delivery, and before the milk threatens. The effect is to superinduce the flow of milk to the nipple, from which it freely and profusely flows, in no case requiring the application of stimulants to induce its discharge, and, by keeping the breasts in constant moisture, effectually prevents hardness by coagulation of milk. In ten days or thereabout the plasters can be taken off without inconvenience.

It is not too much to say that broken or inflamed breasts are impossible when this precautionary mode of treatment is adopted, as it has, in every instance, where it has been tested upon those who before were invariably afflicted with broken breasts, been attended with most triumphant success; and it has thus been put to the test in more than fifty instances to the writer's personal knowledge. In communicating this important fact, therefore, he does so with the most thorough confidence that he is conducing to the amelioration of much suffering, and without assuming that this may not be known to others, he can only say that he has not met with any mention of it in any works to which he has had access. Should those, therefore, into whose hands this work may fall have a wife, or a relation, or a neighbor, who, heretofore, have been afflicted with inflamed or broken breasts, they would have it in their power to ameliorate, nay, prevent much suffering, which to the author of these lines will be a source of heartfelt satisfaction.

MANAGEMENT OF CHILDREN.

It is during infancy that the foundation of a good constitution is generally laid, and it is therefore, important that parents be taught the best method of managing their offspring, in order to preserve their health. Great ignorance is manifested on this subject; it is owing to this that so many children sicken and die: and, furthermore, it is in consequence of this ignorance in our forefathers that the present generation have become so weak, sickly, and effeminate; and most of these evils may be imputed to errors in diet, regimen, *mineral* and *depletive* agents, &c. We have departed from the simplicity of nature, and we must, of course, suffer the penalty.

1*st. On Diet.*—If the mother or nurse has enough of milk, the child will need little or no food for the third or fourth month. It will then be proper to give it a little of some food that is easy of digestion once or twice a day; this will ease the mother, will accustom the child by degrees to take food, and will render the weaning both less difficult and less dangerous. All great and sudden transitions are to be avoided in nursing; for this purpose the food of children ought not only to be simple, but to resemble as nearly as possible the properties of milk: indeed, milk itself should make a principal part of their food, not only before they are weaned, but for some time after.

Next to milk we would recommend good bread, which may be given to a child as soon as it shows an inclination to chew; and it may at all times be allowed as much as it will eat. The very chewing of bread will promote the cutting of the teeth and the discharge of saliva, while, by mixing with the nurse's milk in the stomach, it will afford an excellent nourishment.

Many are in the habit of pouring down various liquids and mixtures made of rich substances, and so much sweetened that the tender organs of digestion are impaired, and acidity and bowel diseases follow; articles of this nature should be avoided: no food, except the milk of the mother, should be given, unless absolutely necessary; nature has designated this liquid exclusively for the nourishment of the infant, and, indeed, we may say, for children.

There is another precaution to be observed, which is, "never to put an infant to a wet-nurse if it can possibly be avoided;" such persons are generally strangers, and they often communicate the most loathsome and fatal diseases; besides, their milk is often rendered unwholesome by age or other causes: this is a very unnatural practice.

The milk of the mother, then, should constitute the only food of the infant, except in cases of disease, when it becomes necessary to obtain a wet-nurse, or bring up the children on the bottle, which can be done very easily.

We attended a lady who was almost covered with a *herpetic complaint*, or the *salt rheum*, and that, too, when her child was born. She was treated and cured her of the complaint. The infant was fed on milk, by introducing a silver tube into a bottle containing it.

We never knew a child so quiet and free from pain; as much so as any offspring of the brute creation, which are free from it merely by following nature or instinct, which never errs. The milk should be of the best quality, and, if possible, of the same cow.

Now, it appears to us, that if females imitated these animals, were to live on vegetable instead of animal food, and drink nothing but water, they would not only bring forth as easy as the Indians or these animals, but their offspring would be free from pain, and perhaps be as exempt from sickness. Would not this course produce a revolution in our habits, health, and in the practice of medicine? In the present diseased state of society it might require a long time to bring about a change in the system; but an immediate benefit would follow by adopting these physiological principles. Do not these facts open a new field of investigation and improvement?

Is it not notorious that some infants are crying a great portion of their time in consequence of pain? and is it natural, or can there be any other cause, except the poison communicated to it, through the medium of the blood, before and after it is born; or the disease may proceed from the impurity of the mother's milk, occasioned by errors in diet? It is self-evident that it is so, from the fact that animals are free from these symptoms.

Can there be any other cause why so many children are in distress from birth, and generally die young, or continue weak and sickly all their lives? There must be a reformation in the habits, taste, and education of modern females. Many mothers are as ignorant, when they have brought a child into the world, of what is to be done for it as the infant itself.

Says Combe: "The leading error in the rearing of the young, I must again repeat, is *over-feeding*, an error serious in itself, but which may easily be avoided by the parent yielding only to the indications of appetite, and administering food slowly and in small quantities at a time. By no other means can the colics, and bowel-complaints, and irritability of the nervous system, so common in infancy, be effectually prevented, and strength and healthy nutrition be secured. Nature never meant the infant stomach to be converted into a receptacle for laxatives, carminatives, antacids, spicy stimulants and astringents; and when these become necessary, we may rest assured that there is something faulty in our management, however perfect it may seem to ourselves. The only exception is where the child is defectively constituted, and then, of course, it may fail to thrive under the best measures which can be advised for its relief.

"Another cause of infantile indigestion, and which is too much overlooked through ignorance of its importance, is *vitiation of the quality of the milk*, caused by imprudence, neglect, or anxiety on the part of the mother The extent to which this cause operates in inducing irritation and suffering in the child, is not generally understood ; and, accordingly, it is not unusual for mothers to display as much indifference to health, regimen, and tranquillity of mind during nursing, as if the milky secretion, and all other bodily functions, were independent of every external and corporeal influence. Healthy, nourishing, and digestible milk can proceed only from a healthy and well-constituted parent; and it is against nature to expect that, if the mother impairs her health and digestion by improper diet, neglect of exercise, impure air, or unruly passions, she can, nevertheless, provide a wholesome and uncontaminated fluid, as if she were exemplary in her observance of all the laws of health.

"It is no new or uncertain doctrine, that the quality of the mother's milk is affected by her own health and conduct, and that in its turn it directly affects the health of the nursling. Even medicines given to the parent act upon the child through the medium of the milk; and a sudden fit of anger, or other violent mental emotion, has not unfrequently been observed to change the quality of the fluid so much as to produce purging and gripes in the child. Care and anxiety in like manner, exert a most pernicious influence, and not only diminish the quantity, but vitiate the quality of the milk.

"It is a common mistake to suppose that, because a woman is nursing, she ought, therefore, to live very fully, and to add an allowance of wine, porter, or other fermented liquor, to her usual diet. The only result of this plan is to cause an unnatural degree of fullness in the system, which places the nurse on the brink of disease, and which of itself frequently puts a stop to, instead of increasing, the secretion of the milk. The health and usefulness of country nurses are often utterly ruined by their transplantation into the families of rich and luxurious employers. Accustomed at home to constant bodily exertion, exposure to the air, and a moderate supply of the plainest food, they live in the enjoyment of the best health, and constitute excellent nurses. But the moment they are transplanted from their proper sphere, their habits and mode of life undergo an unfavourable change. Having no longer any laborious duties to perform or any daily exposure to encounter, they become plethoric and indolent; and as they are at the same time too well fed, the digestive functions become impaired, the system speedily participates in the disorder, and the milk, which was at first bland, nourishing, and plentiful now becomes heating and insufficient, and sometimes even stops altogether."

Cocoa shells, made precisely like coffee, make a very pleasant and nutritious drink for nursing females.

Weaning.—"Diet for infants after weaning may be pure milk, two parts, water, one part; slightly sweetened. This," says Combe, "makes the nearest approach to the nature of the mother's milk, and, therefore, is more suitable than any preparation of milk and flour, or any other that can be given." A child, as a general rule, one year old, ought to be gradually weaned, and the appearance of the teeth shows the propriety of giving food a little more substantial than milk. Bread a day old, mixed with milk and sweetened, may be given in connexion with nursing. Gruel, arrow-root, plain bread, Indian and rice puddings as they grow older, and subsequently bread and butter, thickened milk, hasty pudding or Indian, potatoes, an vegetables. Not a particle of flesh should ever be given. By the use of meat the system becomes excited, and diseases of irritation are apt to be produced, which impede nutrition, and lead ultimately to the production of scrofula and other organic changes in the glands and bowels, and not unfrequently also in the brain and lungs. In these instances the child generally eats heartily, but, nevertheless, continues thin, and is subject to frequent flushing and irregularity of the bowels, headache, and restlessness. His mind partakes of the general irritability of the system, and peevish impatience takes the place of the placid good humour natural to healthy childhood. In this state the ordinary diseases of infancy—measles, scarlet fever, and hooping-cough—are often attended with an unusual and dangerous degree of constitutional disturbance; and when inflammation takes place it is borne with difficulty, and the system does not easily rally; or the digestive organs become irritated, and the various secretions immediately connected with digestion are diminished, especially the biliary secretion. Constipation of the bowels soon follows; congestion of the hepatic and abdominal veins succeeds, and is followed by the train of consequences which have already been detailed. In reality the wonder comes to be, not that so many children die, but that so many survive their early mismanagement. A morbid condition of the system arises, extremely favourable to the production of scrofulous, consumptive, dyspeptic, and other diseases, under which, perhaps, the infant sinks; and yet, strange to state, parents will stuff their children with flesh and grease two or three times a day.

Says Combe, "One of the most pernicious habits in which children can be indulged is that of almost incessant eating. Many mothers encourage it from the facility with which, for a time, the offer of 'something nice' procures peace. Even from infancy the child ought to be gradually accustomed to eat only when hungry, and when food is really required. After two years of age an interval of four hours between meals, will rarely be more than enough; and to give biscuit, fruit, or bread, in the meantime, is just subtracting from the digestive power of the stomach. Like almost every organ of the body, the stomach requires a period of repose after the labour of digestion; and accordingly, in the healthy state, the sensation of appetite never returns till it has been for some time empty. To give food sooner, therefore, is analogous to making a weary traveller walk on without the refreshment of a halt."

"When we reflect that the object of digestion is, to furnish materials for the growth of the body, and to supply the waste which the system is constantly undergoing, it must appear self-evident that, if the digestive powers be impaired by disease, by improper quantity or quality of food, or by any other cause, the result must necessarily be the formation of an imperfect chyle, and, conse quently, of imperfect blood. The elements of the blood are derived from the chyle, and, if *it* be vitiated, the blood also must suffer: if the blood be diseased, so must necessarily be all the organs which it supplies; and if the body be thus debilitated, can any wonder be felt that it should no longer be able to resist the action of offending causes which full health alone can withstand?"

Clothing.—Infants and children are often injured by improper clothing. It is customary for some nurses to wrap them in such a quantity as to injure their health; moderation in this respect should be observed, due regard being paid to that which is sufficient to render them comfortable. Infants, when first born, have clothing enough almost to smother them.

Medicine. — Another very reprehensible custom is, to pour down some nauseous drug, such as paregoric, Godfrey's cordial, or some other articles, every time the child begins to cry or is fretful, by which it becomes habituated to the use of opium, and makes it necessary to increase the dose in order to produce the same effect.

Another injurious practice is to give frequently worm lozenges (the basis of which is calomel or mercury) upon any attack of illness, under the impression that the disorder is occasioned by worms. By this imprudent course both the health and life of the child are endangered. Therefore those who wish to bring up their children in a healthy condition must avoid these evils, and be content to follow the simple path of nature and common sense.

Few things tend more to the destruction f children than drenching them with drugs Medicine may be *sometimes* necessary for children; but that it injures them ten times for once it does them good, I will venture to assert. A nurse or mother, the moment her child seems to ail anything, runs immediately to the doctor or the apothecary, who throws in his powders, pills and potions, till the poor infant is poisoned; when the child might have been restored to perfect health by a change of diet, air, exercise, clothing, or some very easy and simple means.

Care must be taken to keep the bowels regular, which may be effected in most cases by the milk of the mother alone. Most of the complaints in children arise from flatulence or wind; to remove which give common catnip or fennel seed tea, let them drink it freely, and let the mother regulate her diet.

When children complain of pain in the stomach and bowels, it may be necessary sometimes to give a moderate dose of vegetable physic; *senna* and *manna* is very good after the operation of physic let the diet b attended to. Green fruit must be avoided. and whatever is hard of digestion. The feet should be often bathed in warm water the bowels must be fomented with bitter herbs, and it is also necessary to give the child sufficient exercise in the open air.

Bathing should never be neglected, as it contributes much to health. Many complaints of the skin and the system are caused by the neglect of this practice. Filth collects on the surface, obstructs perspiration, which retains morbid humors, and which are thrown upon some of the internal organs and create irritation. Is it not owing to this that infants fret and cry so much? Daily bathe with tepid water; this is also good for galling, chafing, excoriations, &c.

Pure Air and Exercise.—This is very necessary; impure and confined air with the want of exercise, causes disease; and hence children in cities are more pale, feeble, and sickly than those who live in the country and breathe pure air and play in the dirt. Confining children at home, in low, confined, dirty houses, cellars, and in school-rooms, is pernicious; also crowding too many in sleeping-rooms. When children are confined in small apartments, the air not only becomes unwholesome, but the heat relaxes their solids, renders them delicate, and disposes them to colds and many other disorders. Nor is the custom of wrapping them too close in cradles less pernicious. One would think that nurses were afraid lest children should suffer by breathing free air, as many of them actually cover the child's face while asleep, and others wrap a covering over the whole cradle, by which means the child is forced to breathe the same air over and over all the time it sleeps. Children, therefore, must have as much *exercise* and *air* as possible, and should be employed in something useful and interesting.

Again; "The premature exertion of intellect to which the mind is stimulated at our schools, by the constant emulation and vanity, far from strengthening, tends to impair the health and tone of the brain, and of all the organs depending on it; and hence we rarely perceive the genius of the school manifesting in future years any of the superiority which attracted attention in early life"

BARRENNESS.

STERILITY proceeds from either a temporary or permanent incapability of conceiving or retaining the embryo, till it acquires a form. The causes producing this incapability, may consist in some malformation or deficiency of the womb, or its appendages, which cannot always be discovered during life, or in merely a weakness in the action of the womb. This last is by far the most frequent cause, and it is occasioned by local weakness of the womb, or general affections of the whole system; and is marked usually by an obstruction, deficiency, or redundancy of the menstrual evacuation, or by the complaint termed female weakness.

It may be considered as highly probable, that the absence of the capacity to be impregnated, will sometimes depend upon the imperfect condition of either the uterus itselt or of the ovaries. If the former, it may con sist in some derangement of the secreting surface of this organ; for, though there may be a regular discharge of a colored fluid, and this so nearly resembling the perfect secretion as to deceive the senses, it may yet want an essential condition or qualitv and thus entail barrenness—hence, all women are not fruitful who may have a regular catamenial discharge; though, as far as can be determined by appearances, this discharge is every way healthy, and at the same time, the ovaries free from fault.

If it depend upon an imperfection of the ovaria, it may not, perhaps, admit of relief. The diseases of the ovaria may consist, 1st, in their imperfect development; 2dly, in derangement of structure; 3dly, in a want of a healthy organization of the ova themselves. Now, either of these conditions of the ovaria may be so complete as to altogether destroy their influence upon the secreting surface of the uterus; the catamenial discharge may, therefore, continue, with all due regularity, and yet the woman may be barren; and, hence, this discharge cannot be considered, rigidly, as a constant sign of fertility.

Yet it may be safely admitted, as a genera rule, that women who menstruate regularly without pain, or the expulsion of coagula, or false membrane, are fecund; and that the reverse of these conditions is almost sure to be attended with sterility. It may also be observed, that we cannot attach much consequence to the quantity evacuated; for the woman who may evacuate double the quantity of another, is not for this reason more certainly prolific. I have known a number of instances of repeated impregnations, where, as far as could be ascertained, not more than two ounces were habitually evacuated; and this not occupying more than a day and a half, or two days, for its elimination: while, on the contrary, I have known women who were barren, discharge three or four time this quantity; and the fluid bear all the sensible marks of a healthy secretion. From this it would appear, that mere regularity in returns, the elimination of a proper quantity of fluid, and this fluid apparently of a healthy character, do not always declare the woman to be fecund. Yet, when the woman has never menstruated, or when this discharge has altogether ceased, agreeably to the ordinary arrangement of nature, or from disease, she either never becomes impregnated, or ceases to become so, if she ever have been.

We proceed on the principle of rectifying the constitution, where it is injured or weak, and of restoring the menstrual evacuation, to its due and healthy state. The means for effecting these purposes, must depend on the situation of the individual.

Causes.

There are chiefly two states of the constitution productive of those deviations in the action of the womb, which cause barrenness. The first is a state of fulness, and a disposition to obesity.

The person gradually becomes fat and inactive, the menstrual evacuation continue regular for some time; but at last diminishes, and becomes obstructed, or goes to the opposite extreme, and becomes frequent or profuse The patient is either barren or subject to false conceptions. This state is to be rectified by spare or vegetable diet, total abstinence from malt liquor, regular and constant exercise, especially early in the mornings and on horseback, the prudent use of laxatives, and after some time the cold bath. These means will, if persisted in prudently, effect the desired changes; but if pushed to an undue degree, and especially if repeated purgatives, and much vinegar, or great abstinence be resorted to, the health may be completely ruined.

The second state is that of relaxation; the habit is spare, instead of corpulent; the mind lively, and, perhaps, even irritable; the menstrual evacuation either profuse, or it recurs too frequently, and at times clots and shreds are discharged.

This requires a different treatment: the diet, if not unusually nutritive, is at least not to be sparing, the exercise must not be carried the length of fatigue, the cold bath is useful, and strengthening medicines are required.

Such remedies as have been pointed out for the removal of irregularities of the menstrual evacuations, or of the fiuor albus, must be employed when necessary.

There are also certain diseases of the female genital organs, which, when they exist, are found to cause sterility. Polypus in utero is very generally considered to belong to this class; but although the opinion is generally correct, it is not universally true, for it has happened that conception took place notwithstanding the presence of a very large tumor in the uterus. Of this the late Dr. Beatty (Trans. of the Association of Coll. of Phys. in Ireland, vol. 4) has described a very remarkable instance, which occurred in Dublin in the year 1820. The patient was a lady twenty-five years old, who, in consequence of the indisposition of her husband, had left his bed in May, 1819, to which she did not return until August, 1820. In the previous May she first perceived what she termed a "lump in her womb," attended with external swelling and soreness on pressure at the lower part of the abdomen. This swelling was not permanent, but was observed to disappear during the menstrual period. Finding an increase in her unpleasant symptoms, she applied to Dr. Beatty in September, and on the 28th of that month he made an examination per vaginam. The os uteri was found dilated to the size of a dollar, and in its opening was a large dense substance with a regular smooth surface. On the 10th of November, while out in her carriage, she had a moderate discharge of blood from the vagina, and upon examination the parts were found as they were a month before. At two o'clock the following morning she miscarried, the embryo was entire, the membranes not being ruptured: the contained fœtus was about three months old—a period corresponding with the time at which the connubial intercourse had been resumed, and at which she had last menstruated; and just three months after she first experienced uterine uneasiness. The tumor was expelled in six days afterwards by pains resembling labor, the uterus was inverted by its descent, but on separation of the slight attachment between it and the tumor it was easily reduced. The weight of the tumor was found to be nearly four pounds. This lady was delivered of a healthy boy on the 10th of February, 1822. This was an instance of pregnancy during the existence of a tumor of considerable magnitude in the uterus; but we believe it to be an exception to what usually takes place.

Inflammation, suppuration, calculous depositions, cancer, cauliflower excrescence, corroding ulcer, the irritable uterus of Dr. Gooch, and any disease in which the texture of the uterus is much engaged, or with which the constitution sympathizes strongly, are so many obstacles to impregnation, as are diseases of the ovaria, in which the natural structure of these organs is obliterated, and both of them engaged. Leucorrhœa, when profuse, is very often also attended by barrenness; but this is by no means a constant effect, as we have known instances in which this disease existed to a great extent without preventing impregnation.

A question has arisen whether menstruation is necessary in order that a woman shall be prolific; and it is generally stated that women who do not menstruate cannot conceive. (*Paris and Fonblanque*, Med. Jur. vol. i., p. 214.) This is true when applied to those who have never menstruated, but is not in cases that have had even a single monthly discharge. Foderé (Méd. Légale, vol. i., p. 397, ed. 2me) states that, in the first edition of his work, he had maintained that females who do not menstruate are sterile: but he afterwards was obliged to change his opinion, from having observed some patients under his own care enjoying good health without this evacuation, and bearing many children. One of them was a woman thirty-five years old, the mother of five children, the last of which she was suckling. She was in good robust health, and had never menstruated but once at the age of seventeen years. It would appear that a single occurrence of this periodical evacuation is a sufficient indication of generative power; and although irregularity in subsequent years is frequently attended by sterility, it is not to be taken as an absolute cause of it. There is a form of dysmenorrhœa described by Dr. Denman (Denman's Midwifery, 6th edit., p. 90), and Dr. Dewees (Dewees' Midwifery, p. 154) of Philadelphia, which both these authors state to be produc tive of barrenness. The striking peculiarity in this disease is the formation of an adventitious membrane in the uterus, which is expelled after severe and protracted suffering at each menstrual period. This membrane is sometimes thrown off in pieces, and a others entire, at which time it bears the strongest resemblance to the decidua, so much so that, when it occurs in unmarried females, it may and sometimes does give rise to most painful suspicions. There is a preparation in the museum of the College of Surgeons, Dublin, of an entire membrane of this kind, which might deceive the most experienced eye. Morgagni relates a very remarkable instance in which pregnancy occurred during the existence of the habit just described, but it is probable that there was a suspension of the disease for a time in that case, when the capability of conceiving might exist.

It is well known that instances have happened in which persons have lived for years in unfruitful matrimony, and being after divorce remarried, have both had children. This is a fact which in the present state of our knowledge we are not able satisfactorily to explain, and we will not delay the reader by offering any speculative opinion upon it.

Treatment.

The treatment of impotence and sterility must be influenced by the causes from which they spring, some of which are incurable, whilst others may be removed by appropriate remedies. Those cases which depend upon congenital deficiency of the penis, testicles, vagina, uterus, Fallopian tubes, or ovaria, belong to the former; but we have seen that some of those arising from malformation and disease of these parts are susceptible of cure. Such are phymosis, adhesion of the prepuce to the glands with diminution of the orifice of the urethra, priapism, partial paralysis, strictures in the urethra, diseases of the neighbouring parts, contracted vagina, occlusion of the mouth of this canal by adhesion of the labia, or by a dense hymen, prolapsus and procidentia uteri, polypus in utero, leucorrhœa, dysmenorrhœa: all these are more or less capable of removal either by operation or general treatment.

By persisting carefully in a proper plan, sterility may at length be frequently removed. There are many instances of women bearing children, after having been several years barren.

Various remedies have been recommended for the cure of barrenness, among which tincture of cantharides is the most prominent, but its effects being evanescent, are invariably succeeded by lassitude and debility, and therefore can be attended with no good results. The various preparations of sassafras and sarsaparilla are useless and not in the least calculated to reach the nature of the case. The specific known as the most successful in curing sterility or barrenness—and it has certainly performed wonderful cures—is the celebrated Morand's preparation, called "Morand's Elixir," which appears to be specially adapted to give tone and healthiness to the generative functions, for the discovery of which, he received a handsome donation from the French government, as also frequently rewarded by the liberality of private individuals, who have realized their fond wishes by his discovery.

Its effects, it is said, are so wonderful upon the general health, and particularly upon the generative functions, that a medical writer of some note says that he has recommended its use in several instances, and, with one single exception (a case of malformation), with invariable success. He says:

"I was acquainted with a very worthy married couple whose life was, if not embittered, at least unhappy, because of their having no offspring. They were of respectable and influential standing, possessed of property, surrounded by friends and relatives, were then married nearly ten years, and desirous only of having children to make them happy. Physicians were consulted without success, because physicians mostly look upon sterility as incurable.

"About this time I visited a patient who had been married about seven years without having children, who was affected with fluor albus (whites), and was using 'Morand's

Elixir,' by my recommendation, to eradicate this weakening complaint from the system. This lady having been married seven years, as I before observed, without offspring, had nearly resigned herself to a conviction that she was destined to have none. In recommending 'Morand's Elixir,' I had the fullest confidence that it would accomplish a thorough cure of her complaint, because I had often used it in my practice, and with invariable success, but I had neither hope nor expectation of its ability to remove what I then considered confirmed sterility, or barrenness, as I then gave no credence to the various marvellous properties it was alleged to possess, classing it merely among the impositions of the day. The lady continued its use, and I found her health evidently and perceptibly improve. The fluor albus entirely disappeared and her health was restored. Under pretence that she derived great benefit from it she still continued its use, however, and to my utter surprise, as well as the great joy of her husband, four months after she commenced its use, she became pregnant, and in due time was delivered of a fine, fat, healthy daughter, and had two more children in close succession after.*

* That barrenness, in most cases, arises from some defect or obstruction, susceptible of cure, the fact, that those who for a number of years have had no children, when once becoming pregnant—the defect or obstruction being eradicated—have children in close succession, may be adduced as almost conclusive proof.

"The lady being of the most pure and irreproachable character, it may well be supposed that it gave me the greatest confidence in recommending this truly wonderful 'Elixir,' in like cases. When, therefore, I was consulted by the husband of the lady first mentioned, I did not hesitate to recommend 'Morand's Elixir.' and informing him of its effect in the case described. My advice was followed. In due course of time this worthy couple had their fondest wishes realized. Since which time they also have had several children. Their gratitude to me for recommending its use, was unbounded. My confidence in the virtues of 'Morand's Elixir,' was confirmed, and I have heard of its success in other instances. Indeed, I am convinced, that if the case is curable, 'Morand's Elixir' is infallible."

It has attained a pre-eminent celebrity in France, Germany, on the continent of Europe generally, as well as in England, for its unexampled success in removing general debility, weakness, physical imbecility and *supposed* barrenness (for judging from the astonishing results of 'Morand's Elixir,' it is denied that it really exists). The truly wonderful effect of the "Morand's Elixir," has now established the fact that most, if not all, *supposed natural* incurable defects, are *only artificial* ones, within the powers of the skill and scientific combination of the virtues and essences of the most nourishing, strengthening and invigorating fruits and plants of Italy to remove Its action is not sudden and ephemeral, leaving the system but the more debilitated by reason of the previous unnatural excitement, but is gentle and gradual, by degrees displacing the latent causes affecting the body, strengthening and invigorating the generative functions, cheering the mind, enlivening the spirits, engendering a free, full and healthy circulation, and thus arousing the sexual feelings.

Great and surprising as are the results of the skilful and scientific combination in the composition of "Morand's Elixir," it is not idly pretended that without any reference to the circumstances of each individual case of supposed barrenness, it will, unaided and unassisted, in a few weeks, remove deep seated and obstinate cases of unfruitfulness—causes which had been growing, strengthening and fastening for years. Far from it. The absurdity of such pretence is manifest on the face of it. Assistants, in many instances, must be resorted to for successful treatment, in respect to diet, clothing, occupation, &c. Instant and immediate relief is neither to be expected nor practicable; and even if practicable would lead to the most injurious results, aggravating instead of relieving. A remedy, therefore, to be permanent, must be gradual to an almost imperceptible degree, slowly but surely removing the stagnant humors and impure secretions, by the searching and penetrating virtues of the "Elixir," systematically purging the system of those dormant and inactive particles, which frustrate the action of the generative functions, and thus dislodging the cause of unfruitfulness. It may take some time ere this is accomplished; but, by a proper perseverance in the course marked out, success, sooner or later, is inevitable. Thousands who had imagined themselves irretrievably doomed to descend to the grave unpitied and unmourned by interesting and affectionate children have, by the use of "Morand's Elixir," been blessed with offspring to love and adore in infancy and youth, and to look to for comfort and solace in old age.

In all cases of incontinence of urine, fluor albus, gleet, painful and difficult menstruation, incipient stages of consumption, languor, debility, night sweats and wakefulness, it is surprisingly efficient and certain. Its chief and great celebrity, however, in eradicating every symptom of that state of the functions superinducing barrenness or sterility, is too well established to require comment. Indeed, such has been its success, as to make it doubtful that what is usually termed barrenness in fact exists, since by the use of this wonderful remedy, properly persevered in, a cure has in all cases been effected, and what had been supposed incurable natural defects proved to be only some deranged state of the functions.

As there are many who pine and grieve

for children—who feel desolate and lonely without the enlivening and cheering influence of children around the domestic hearth, the author does not deem it inappropriate or out of place to present this celebrated specific for the consideration of those to whom it might prove a great blessing. He has taken its Agency for the United States, at his Office, 129 Liberty-street. Letters must be post-paid and addressed to Box "1224," New-York City.

Price Five Dollars,

And can be forwarded by mail or express, with full directions.

CONCLUDING REMARKS.

In conclusion, the author of this work trusts that it may prove an invaluable blessing as well to the unmarried as married, to those in affluence as well as to those in penury. To the matured woman in the full enjoyment of the elasticity and vigor of health, its pages direct how to retain that precious boon. To the weak, sickly, debilitated one, it lays bare the causes of her malady, and points out the remedy. To the young female about blooming into maturity—that critical juncture, involving her future health and welfare, its pages reveal the shoals and quicksands, surrounding her on all sides, and the necessary steps to avoid them. To the female already suffering from various complaints, arising either from retention or stoppage of the menses, their irregularity, or too profuse flow, the means of a thorough and effectual cure are pointed out. To the woman suffering in health from a too rapid increase of family, the perusal of these pages shows that pregnancy can and should, under some circumstances, be prevented. To those unblessed with children, from a supposed existence of barrenness, the indubitable facts herein contained, demonstrate that by following certain suggestions the result may not be *fruitless.*

In short, in all the relations of life in which a female can be placed, whether as a daughter, a wife, or a mother—whether in the enjoyment of good, or suffering under ill-health—whether physically formed capable of enduring the various trials imposed upon her by nature, or whether mal-formed or physically incapable to endure them, this little book is one that no female having a regard for her own welfare, or that of her husband or children, will be without.

Spotted something that isn't quite right?

Let us know and we'll fix it for future reprints.
And as a thank you for your diligence, we'll
send you a free Sothis book of your choice.

publisher@sothis.press

This page intentionally left blank

Made in the USA
Monee, IL
05 November 2026

67979973R00156